ATKINS DIET RECIPES

The Atkins and Vegan-friendly Ketogenic Guide for Weight Loss

(Quick Start Guide for the Atkins Diet)

William Olvera

Published by Alex Howard

© **William Olvera**

All Rights Reserved

Atkins Diet Recipes: The Atkins and Vegan-friendly Ketogenic Guide for Weight Loss (Quick Start Guide for the Atkins Diet)

ISBN 978-1-990169-62-5

All rights reserved. No part of this guide may be reproduced in any form without permission in writing from the publisher except in the case of brief quotations embodied in critical articles or reviews.

Legal & Disclaimer

The information contained in this book is not designed to replace or take the place of any form of medicine or professional medical advice. The information in this book has been provided for educational and entertainment purposes only.

The information contained in this book has been compiled from sources deemed reliable, and it is accurate to the best of the Author's knowledge; however, the Author cannot guarantee its accuracy and validity and cannot be held liable for any errors or omissions. Changes are periodically made to this book. You must consult your doctor or get professional medical advice before using any of the suggested remedies, techniques, or information in this book.

Table of contents

Part 1 1
Introduction 2
Chapter 1: Getting Started With Atkins Diet 3
What Is The Atkins Diet 3
Logic Behind Atkins Diet 3
Tips To Follow Dr. Atkins' Diet 3
Chapter 2: Red Meat 5
Meat & Potato Bake 5
Smothered Hash Browns 5
Cheese Balls 6
Cheesy Sausage Balls 6
Steak And Eggs 7
Reuben Dip 7
Stuffed Peppers 8
Cabbage With Beef 9
Juicy Lucy Sliders 9
Chapter 3: Chicken 11
Crispy Wings 11
Chicken Nuggets 11
Buffalo Chicken 12
Chicken Salad 12

Chicken Broccoli Soup 13

Loaded Baked Chicken 14

Spicy Chicken Thighs 14

Shirataki Chicken Alfredo 15

Chicken Cordon Bleu Casserole 16

Chapter 4: Sea Food 17

Tuna Salad 17

Stuffed And Wrapped Shrimp 17

Quick Steamed Red Snapper 18

Simple Shrimp Dip 18

Iceberg Salad With Shrimp 19

Shrimp And Mushroom Cowder 20

Cod With Oregano 21

Ritz Fish 21

Lori's Oil Poached Fish 22

Chapter 5 - Desserts 23

The Ultimate Punch 23

Chocolate Energy Bars 23

Chocolate Strawberry Mousse 24

Eggnog 25

Coffee Cooler 25

Homemade Whipped Cream 26

Coconut Macaroons 26

Chocolate Hearts 27

Mint Chocolate Chip Ice Cream 28

Almond Cakes 28

Almond Bun Pizza 30

Chapter 6 - Others 31

Western Scrambled Eggs 31

Brussels Sprout Burgers 31

Chorizo Breakfast Casserole 32

Bacon Hash 33

Deep Fried Eggs 34

Baked Eggs 34

Deviled Egg Chicks 35

Atkins Lightly Spicy Turnip Fries 36

Almond Buns 36

Taco Salad 37

Tomato-Mozzarella Stacks 38

Pita Pizza 38

Chicken Broccoli Soup 39

Roasted Duck 39

Bourbon Glazed Ham 40

Bacon Cheddar Cauliflower Soup 41

Keto Dip 42

Fried Broccoli 43

Spinach Crap 43

Spicy Fried Brussels Sprouts 44

Creamy Cheesy Spinach 44

Mashed Cauliflower 44

Valentine's Day Eggs For Two – Phase 1 46

Valentine's Day Crab Cakes – Phase 1 46

Valentine's Day Heart-Y Pot Pies – Phase 3 47

Valentine's Day Chococado Smoothies – Phase 2 48

St. Patrick's Day Green Frittata – Phase 1 49

St. Patrick's Corned Beef And Cabbage Hash – Phase 2 50

St. Paddy's Day Dinner Salad – Phase 1 50

St. Patrick's Green Smoothie – Phase 4 51

Mardi Gras Faux Beignets – Phase 4 52

Mardi Gras Muffalettas – Phase 4 53

Mardi Gras Seafood Gumbo – Phase 2 53

Mardi Gras King Cake Minis – Phase 3 55

Easter Egg Muffins – Phase 1 56

Easter Cauli-Egg Salad – Phase 2 57

Easter Roasted Brisket – Phase 3 57

Easter Carrot Cottontails – Phase 3 58

Fourth Of July Cheesy Apple Strudel – Phase 4 59

Fourth Of July Cbt Snacks – Phase 1 60

Fourth Of July Spicy Chicken Wraps – Phase 4 60

Fourth Of July Red, White, And Berries – Phase 3 61

Memorial/Veterans Day Biscuits & Gravy – Phase 4 62

Memorial/Veterans Day Game Hens - Phase 3 63

Memorial/Veterans Day No-Tortilla Fajitas – Phase 1 64

Memorial/Veterans Day Cheesecake Flags – Phase 3 65

Halloween Spookyface Fruits – Phase 4 67

Halloween Itsy Bitsy Spiders – Phase 1 67

Halloween Spiced Apple Chicken – Phase 3 68

Halloween Goblin Balls – Phase 4 68

Thanksgiving Flax Muffin – Phase 2 69

Thanksgiving Smoky Green Beans – Phase 4 70

Thanksgiving Stuffed Turkey Omelets – Phase 1 70

Thanksgiving Pumpkin Yogurt – Phase 3 71

Christmas Dreamy Sweet Potatoes – Phase 3 72

Christmas Festive Coleslaw – Phase 1 73

Christmas Apple-Stuffed Pork – Phase 3 73

Christmas Almond Biscotti – Phase 4 74

Part 2 76

Atkins Breakfast Recipes 77

All Purpose Low-Carb Baking Mix 77

Almond And Coconut Muffin In A Minute 78

Almond Muffin In A Minute 79

Almond Protein Pancakes With Blueberries 81

Almond Protein Pancakes 82

Almond-Pineapple Smoothie 83

Almond-Pumpkin Pancakes 84

Almond-Raspberry Smoothie 86

Ancho Macho Chili 87

Apple Muffins With Cinnamon-Pecan Streusel 88

Asian Beef Salad Single Serving 90

Atkins Cinnamon Pie Crust 92

Atkins Cuisine Biscuits 93

Atkins Cuisine Pancakes 95

Atkins Cuisine Pie Crust 96

Atkins Cuisine Waffles 98

Bacon, Avocado And Jack Cheese Omelets With Fresh Salsa . 99

Baked Eggs And Asparagus 101

Basque Eggs With Ham, Tomatoes And Bell Peppers 102

Béchamel Sauce 104

Beef Huevos Rancheros On Canadian Bacon 105

Beef Sautéed With Green Bell Pepper And Onions Topped With Cheese 107

Bell Pepper Rings Filled With Egg And Mozzarella With Fruit 108

Blackberry Smoothie 109

Blueberry Cloud Muffin 110

Breakfast Burrito 112

Breakfast Mexi Peppers 113

Breakfast Sausage Sautéed With Red And Green Bell Peppers 115

Buttermilk Cinnamon Waffles 116

California Breakfast Burrito 117

Canadian Bacon, Cheddar And Tomato Stacks 119

Carrot-Zucchini Latkes 120

Cheddar Omelet With Avocado And Salsa 122

Cheddar Omelet With Sautéed Onions And Shiitake Mushrooms 123

Cheddar Omelet With Sautéed Onions 124

Cheddar Omelet With Sautéed Tomato And Zucchini 125

Cheddar Omelet With Sautéed Watercress 127

Cheddar Omelet With Swiss Chard And Onions 127

Cheese And Spinach Omelet Topped With Avocado And Salsa 129

Cheese Baked Eggs 130

Cheesy Bacon Cloud Muffin 131

Chicken Chorizo And Cauliflower Saute With Cheese And Salsa 132

Chicken-Portobello Broilers 133

Chili Spiced "Tortilla" Wraps 135

Chocolate And Strawberry Smoothie ... 136
Chocolate Cake Donuts ... 137
Chocolate Cloud Muffin ... 139
Chocolate Hazelnut Smoothie ... 140
Chocolate Peanut Butter Smoothie ... 141
Chorizo, Green Chili And Tomato Frittata ... 142
Cinnamon Buns ... 144
Cinnamon Churritos ... 146
Cinnamon Crumb Coffee Cake ... 147
Cinnamon Mini Muffins ... 149
Coconut-Vanilla Shake ... 150
Corned Beef Hash ... 150
Creamy Scrambled Eggs With Dill And Smoked Salmon ... 151
Crunchy Tropical Berry And Almond Breakfast Parfait ... 152
Crustless Broccoli Quiche ... 153
Crustless Pumpkin And Ham Quiche ... 155
Crustless Spinach Quiche ... 156
Double-Chocolate Express Smoothie ... 157
Dutch Baby Baked Pancake ... 157
Eggs And Spinach ... 159
Eggs Scrambled With Asparagus, Bacon And Swiss Cheese 159
Eggs Scrambled With Avocado, Onions And Tomato ... 160
Eggs Scrambled With Cheddar And Swiss Chard ... 161

Eggs Scrambled With Cheddar, Swiss Chard And Canadian Bacon 162

Eggs Scrambled With Feta And Spinach 163

Eggs Scrambled With Sautéed Mushrooms And Zucchini.... 163

Eggs Scrambled With Sautéed Onions And Cheddar Cheese 164

Eggs Scrambled With Zucchini, Cheddar And Sour Cream.. 165

Eggs With Avocado And Salsa With Cantaloupe And Sausage 166

Eggs With Avocado And Salsa 167

Eggs With Avocado And Tomato 167

Eggs With Avocado, Salsa And Turkey Bacon 168

Eggs With Avocado, Tomato And Sausage 169

Eggs With Cheddar, Asparagus, Salsa And Sour Cream...... 169

Farmers Breakfast Soup 170

Fennel, Carrot Hash And Turkey Hash 171

Feta And Red Bell Pepper Omelet 172

Fluffy Flax Waffles With Turkey Sausage 173

Fluffy Flax Waffles 174

French Quesadillas 176

French Toast Casserole 176

French Toast Loaf 178

Frittata Lorraine 179

Garden Frittata 180

Giant Zucchini Pancake 181

Green Bell Pepper Filled With Creamy Eggs And Spinach ... 182

Ham And Cheese Roll-Ups 183

Part 1

Introduction

Atkins is all about consuming scrumptious and nutritious food, a wide range of protein, fruits, leafy and other veggies, whole grains and nuts. Over 50 reports support the low-carb Atkins diet.

The Atkins Diet Recipes is developed to assist you in reducing weight, making use of the Atkins Diet, right from the start. Find out ways to eat healthier foods that will convert your body into a wonderful fat burning machine.

Compared with other Atkins Diet books, Atkins Diet Recipes is the only guidebook developed for busy families. Inside, you will discover full step-by-step Atkins Diet Recipes of red meat, chicken and seafood you can make less than 30 minutes that even most kids with particular taste buds will really like. These recipes are comprehensive with information like carbs and calories, so you can also monitor your calorie consumption.

This crucial book helps make low-carb cooking simpler than ever before. Explained with photographs, it contains 60 recipes for delicious dishes like:

- Cheese Balls
- Shirataki Chicken Alfredo
- Quick Steamed Red Snapper
- Atkins Lightly Spicy Turnip Fries
- The Ultimate Punch and more!

Thanks again for downloading this book, I hope you enjoy it!

Chapter 1: Getting Started With Atkins Diet

What Is The Atkins Diet

The Atkins Diet, basically known as the "Atkins Nutritional Approach", is a low carbohydrate diet publicized by Robert Atkins from a research paper he studies in "The Journal of the American Medical Association" posted by Alfred W. Pennington, named "Weight Reduction", posted in 1958.

Atkins made use of the study to settle his personal obese problem. He afterwards made popular the technique in a set of books, starting with the Dr. Atkins' Diet Revolution in 1972. In his 2nd book, Dr. Atkins' New Diet Revolution (2002), he changed components of the diet but did not change the initial ideas.

Logic Behind Atkins Diet

The concept is that when you significantly reduce carbs, your body converts your fat stores for energy resource. The final result is you burn off body fat, releasing a byproduct known as ketones that you will use for energy. The program is not advised for people with serious kidney illness.

There is fairly a little research on low-carb diets for weight-loss and control of diabetes. Reports demonstrate that low-carb diets are as useful for weight-loss as conventional techniques and will boost cholesterol and triglycerides. But like all diets, it could be complicated to follow for a very long time.

Tips To Follow Dr. Atkins' Diet

Choosing a low-carb diet is a difficult task, definitely. But it will also be very useful and provide the outcomes you have been seeking. Just before you begin Atkins, you should realize some of the primary techniques along with the best way to fight some adverse effects of the diet.

1. Take time to visit your cabinets and fridge to be free from the bad stuff foods.

   Foods to avoid:

   Foods that contain sugar or any kind of sugar, just like honey.

   Foods that contain white flour Hydrogenated fats, also called trans fats

   They are synthetic fats that harm your overall health. The US Government prompts to eat very little trans fat.

2. People encounter a variety of bodily and psychological issues when they are working to stick to the Atkins diet. Even so, if you understand the prospective disadvantages in advance, then you can fight them by taking precautionary actions.

3. Go with Atkins diet products. Atkins International delivers a number of low-carb shakes and protein bars.

4. Make a grocery list of food items to keep available for your new diet plan. Note down good protein resources just like turkey, tuna fish, eggs and chicken breasts. Do not neglect low-carb vegetables, just like lettuce, mushrooms, and cucumbers.

5. Eat frequently. Eat at least after every six hours. You can pick to take possibly 3 meals daily or 5 to 6 small meals. When you eat, be sure to only eat till you come to feel full. Never eat too much.

Chapter 2: Red Meat

Meat & Potato Bake

Ingredients:

2 lbs = ground beef

1/2 cup = steak sauce

4 = medium potatoes (peeled and thinly sliced)

1 cup = shredded cheddar cheese

1 cup = seasoned dry bread crumb

2/3 cup = chopped onion

Directions:

Preheat the oven to 350 °F. Put potatoes in the base of evenly greased baking pot; put to one side. Store 1/4 cup of steak sauce.

Combine leftover 1/4 cup steak sauce with onion, meat and bread crumbs in big basin. Spread lightly on potatoes, pushing tightly to shape hard layer.

Brush with stored steak sauce. Cook in the oven at least 1 hour or till meat mix is fit to be eaten. Add cheese and continue cooking 5 minutes or till cheese is evenly melted.

Let it set 10 minutes prior to serving.

Smothered Hash Browns

Ingredients:

1 can = mushrooms (sliced)

1 lb = stew meat (cut bite size)

1 = green pepper (chopped)

16 ounces = cheddar cheese (shredded)

2 lbs = hash browns

1 = onion (chopped)

Directions:

Heat the oil in big pan. Brown the hash browns until crunchy.

While hash browns are frying, sauté the stew meat in another pan and keep aside.

Fry onions and green peppers until tender.

Put in mushrooms to onions and peppers. Mix in stew meat with onion mix, heat throughout.

Place hash browns on serving platter and drop cheese. Put meat mix on top.

Cheese Balls

Ingredients:

1 package = cheddar cheese

1 package = sausage meat

2 cups = Bisquick

Directions:

Slice cheese and include leftover ingredients into it. Spin mixture to make balls. Cook in the oven at 375 F for 10 minutes.

Cheesy Sausage Balls

Ingredients:

6 oz = Shredded Cheddar cheese

12 oz = Sausage

12 = Cubes Cheddar (Optional)

Directions:

Combine shredded cheese and sausage. Separate into 12 equal parts. Put cube of cheese into the middle of sausage and roll into balls. Chill the sausage balls. Fry at 375 degrees till crunchy.

Steak And Eggs

Ingredients:

15 = Eggs

1 = Onion (270 g)

1 = Pepper (180 g)

4 Lbs = Beef Chuck Shoulder

120 g = Heavy Cream

5 Oz = Cheddar Cheese

Salt, Pepper, Onion Powder, Garlic Powder (to taste)

Directions:

Cut up the peppers and onions.

Fry the peppers and onions till lucid and put to one side. Cook the steak on high heat for 6 minutes or till preferred internal temperature has been reached.

Let steak rest while cooking eggs Combine eggs, cream, and spices in a large bowl. Cook in a non-stick pan, whisking occasionally, until they are no longer runny Add cheese and whisk some more. Combine all the ingredients in a container for breakfast!

Reuben Dip

Ingredients:

1/4 cup = Thousand Island dressing

2 cups = corned beef (shredded cooked)

16 ozs = sauerkraut (drained)

2 cups = Swiss cheese

8 ozs = cream cheese, soften

Directions:

In a crock pot, mix the sauerkraut, cream cheese, Swiss cheese, corned beef and Thousand Island dressing. Cover, and cook on high heat for at least 45 minutes if you're in a rush, low for more time if you're not, or just till hot and cheese is melted. Mix from time to time while cooking.

Stuffed Peppers

Ingredients:

1 = Small Onion

1 = Egg

2 Oz. = Cream Cheese

2 = Quail Eggs

2 = Sausage Links

2 = Green Peppers

1.5 Oz = Parmesan Cheese

Directions:

Begin by removing the covering of the sausage and cooking the sausage into piece

Cut the top of the peppers and eliminate the seeds.

Cut up the tops of the peppers. Cut up the onions as well and cook the peppers and onions together. Chop up Parmesan cheese into tiny pieces.

Mix the onions, peppers, sausage, cheese and cream cheese. Stuff the peppers with the filling and end with a quail egg.

Cook for almost 20 minutes at 400 degrees.

Cabbage With Beef

Ingredients:

1.029 Kg = Green Cabbage

½ = Cup Water

24 oz = Pasta Sauce

24 oz = Ground beef

1 stick = Unsalted Butter

Salt and pepper

Directions:

Begin by removing the outermost coat of cabbage and disposal. Divide into four parts the cabbage and grate in a blender.

Melt butter in a large pan and put in the cabbage as well as water, add salt and pepper. Cover up and cook for almost 12 minutes, moving irregularly.

When the cabbage is cooking, fry the beef and drain it. Include the beef to the cabbage and mix it.

Add in the pasta sauce as well and mix again. Garnish it with cheese.

Juicy Lucy Sliders

Ingredients:

1 = Egg

Onion Powder

8 oz = Cheddar Cheese

Several dashes = Worcestershire Sauce

6 oz = Ground Beef

Garlic

Salt and Pepper

Directions:

Combine the beef, eggs and the spices.

Separate the meat into 1.5 oz patties. Put in ½ oz of cheese to each patty.

Mix two patties to make a burger. Make use of your hands to set the patties together.

Warm some oil on high heat and fry the burgers to your preferred completion stage.

Chapter 3: Chicken

Crispy Wings

Ingredients:
12 = Chicken Wings
4 Tbsp = Red Hot
4 Tbsp = Unsalted Butter

Directions:
Preheat fryer oil to 275. Pat wings down so they are super dry. Fry wings for 14 minutes. Let wings rest until back to room temperature.
Preheat fryer to 375. Pat wings dry. Fry for 6 more minutes or until golden brown and the skin is taut. Optionally, mix together Red Hot and melted butter and toss the wings in the sauce.

Chicken Nuggets

Ingredients:
1 Tbsp = Water
1 = egg
1 = Chicken Breast (Cooked)
½ tsp = Baking Powder
½ Oz. = Grated Parmesan
2 Tbsp = Almond Flour

Directions:
Begin by heating your fryer to 375 degrees.
Cook a chicken breast and then cut into cubes.

Combine the almond flour, grated parmesan, and baking powder.

Include the egg and whip. Include the water and whip again.

Spin the chicken breasts in the batter till they are totally covered, then make use of a fork to put them into the oil.

Be sure that they do not stick to the base. Cook till the batter becomes golden brown, almost 5 minutes.

Buffalo Chicken

Ingredients:
6 = Frozen Chicken Breasts
½ Packet = Hidden Valley Ranch
3 Tbsp = Butter
1 Bottle = Red Hot

Directions:
Place the chicken in the slow cooker. Add the hot sauce on chicken and drop ranch over top.

Cover up and cook on low heat for 5 hours.

Grate, include butter, and cook on low heat for nearly 1 hour open.

Chicken Salad

Ingredients:
¾ Cup = Mayo
125 g = Celery
20 g = Green Onions

4 = Chicken Breasts
3 = Hardboiled Eggs
¾ Cup = Sugar Free Sweet Relish
105 g = Green peppers

Directions:

Pre-heat oven to 350 degrees! Put in chicken to an oven proof pan with a cover. Put in cream to cover chicken.

Cook for 50 minutes till chicken is done.

Place 3 eggs into a pan and cover up with water let it boil and cook for 15 minutes when boiling.

When chicken is cooking, cut up the celery, peppers and onions and let chicken cool and cut.

Mix all ingredients into large pot. Cut the eggs and mix in. Divide the mixture into 6 boxes.

Chicken Broccoli Soup

Ingredients:

12 oz = Cheddar Cheese, Shredded
1 Can = Chicken Broth
8 = Chicken Thighs
1.5 cups = Heavy Cream
4 Slices = Bacon
780 g = Broccoli
Salt, pepper, garlic powder and onion powder (To Taste)

Directions:

Pre-heat oven to 350 degrees! Put chicken thighs in saucepan with a lid, add spices, and also water.

When chicken is cooking, sauté 4 slices of bacon. Fry Broccoli as well in bacon grease, and mash the broccoli as much as possible with spatula.

As chicken is ready and cooled, put into container. Put in broccoli and bacon, combine over medium heat. Include cheese, heavy cream and broth. Heat till thickened.

Loaded Baked Chicken

Ingredients:
3 = Green Onions
4 Oz. = Cheddar Cheese
4 Oz. = Ranch Dressing
4 = Chicken Breasts
1 Oz. = Soy Sauce
4 = Bacon Strips

Directions:
Heat the pan with some oil on high heat.

Fry chicken breasts, turning half way, till inner temperature reaches 165, most likely 10-15 minutes.

When chicken is cooking, arrange bacon bits by frying then breakup.

Chop up 3 green onion stalks as well.

Transfer chicken in a baking plate and top with soy sauce, ranch, bacon, green onions and cheese in given order.

Broil on high heat till the cheese melts, nearly 3-4 minutes.

Spicy Chicken Thighs

Ingredients:

1 = Small Onion

3 Tbsp = Lime Juice

2 Tbsp = Chili Garlic Sauce

8 = Chicken Thighs

Salt and Pepper to taste

Directions:

Sprinkle Salt and pepper to the chicken thighs on both sides.

Mix the lime juice and chili sauce in a large basin. Put in the onions and chicken to the basin and combine. Shift to an oven safe pan and cook for 35 minutes at 400 degrees or till the inner temperature becomes 180 degrees.

Shirataki Chicken Alfredo

Ingredients:

2 Large = Chicken breast

2 8 Oz. Packages = Noodles

1 Jar = Alfredo Sauce

300 g = Spinach

2 Tbsp = Minced Garlic

Parmesan Cheese

Salt and pepper

Directions:

Dice the chicken breasts and sauté, and then drain it. Thaw the frozen spinach in a pot till cooked. Put in the sauce to the spinach and include salt, pepper and garlic.

Include chicken to sauce. Wash noodles then pan fry them. Mix sauce with noodles and serve with grated Parmesan Cheese.

Chicken Cordon Bleu Casserole

Ingredients:
11 oz = Jarhlsberg Swiss cheese
53 oz = Chicken (boneless)
1 Cup = Heavy Whipping Cream
300 g = Ham Steak
1 cup = Cream Cheese
Salt, Pepper,
Garlic Powder

Directions:
Cut up chicken into cubes, extend on base of saucepan.
Add Salt, pepper and garlic powder to the chicken.
Chop up the ham into cubes and add on top of chicken. Grate Swiss cheese and put over mixtures.
Warm the cream cheese in the microwave, and then put in the cream and combine, transfer over casserole. Mix up the dish.
Bake at 350 degrees for 40 minutes.

Chapter 4: Sea Food

Tuna Salad

Ingredients:

7 Containers = Tuna in Water Strained

¾ Cup = Mayo

25 g = Green Onion

160 g = Celery

¾ Cup = Sugar Free Relish

3 = Hard boiled Eggs

140 g = Green Pepper

Directions:

Hard boil the eggs. Open tuna and pull out the water. Crumble tuna in a basin. Include all ingredients and mix as well.

Stuffed And Wrapped Shrimp

Ingredients:

1.5 Lbs = Large, (cooked and peeled shrimp)

15 slices = Bacon

1 Tbsp = Pepper

15 = Jalapeno Slices

¼ tsp = Cayenne Pepper

5 Slices = Cheddar Cheese

1 Tbsp = Garlic Powder

1 Tbsp = Paprika

Directions:

If your shrimp is frozen, melt them in water.

Combine the four dry ingredients in a basin.

Dry the thawed and peeled shrimp and combine with ¾ of the spice mixture.

Slice the shrimp and put half a jalapeno slice and a little cheese into the opening.

Slice bacon in half and wrap the shrimp; try and cover it such that the start and end both are close to a center.

Skewer the shrimp. Grill till the bacon is crunchy.

Quick Steamed Red Snapper

Ingredients:

1 lb = red snapper fillet

1 = garlic clove (minced)

1 tablespoon = light soy sauce

1/8 teaspoon = black pepper

1 tablespoon = sugar

1 teaspoon = fresh ginger, finely grated

1/8 teaspoon = salt

Directions:

Mix up ginger, soy sauce, sugar, garlic, salt and pepper.

Place fish on hot stand. Cover fish with soy ginger mixture. Put stand over boiling water and co

Steam it for 10 minutes. Brush occasionally with soy ginger mixture.

Simple Shrimp Dip

Ingredients:

2 = green onions

4 ounces = seafood cocktail sauce

8 ounces = light cream cheese (soften)

8 ounces = mayonnaise

1/2 lb = baby shrimp

Directions:

Cut up green onions and keep aside. Combine cream cheese and mayonnaise and set in serving dish. Wash off shrimp and put over mixture. On top of shrimp add cocktail sauce. Garnish with green onions.

Iceberg Salad With Shrimp

Ingredients:

1 cup = small shrimp

1 head = iceberg lettuce

2 tablespoons = lemon zest

1/2 cup = seafood cocktail sauce, prepared

3 tablespoons = chives (chopped)

3 drops = hot sauce

1 = lemon (juiced)

1/4 cup = mayonnaise

1/2 teaspoon = salt

1/4 teaspoon = pepper

Directions:

Take away core out of lettuce head. Cut up the head of lettuce end-to-end. Mix lemon juice, cocktail sauce, mayo, hot sauce and zest.

Mix shrimp into dressing and spread it lightly down over quartered lettuce.

Add salt and pepper to salads and spread chives over the salads and eat.

Shrimp And Mushroom Cowder

Ingredients:
1/2 cup = whipping cream
1/4 cup = all-purpose flour
1/2 lb = shrimp (cooked)
1/2 lb = mushroom (sliced)
1/2 cup = wine (dry white)
1/2 = thyme leaves (dried)
1/2 teaspoon = dill
1 = onion (chopped)
2 tablespoons = butter
2 cups = fish stock
1/4 teaspoon = salt
1/4 teaspoon = mace

Directions:
Buy cleaned shrimp and drain well.

Fry mushrooms and onion in butter for almost 2 minute or till onion is soft. Mix in flour.

Fry for 1 minute additionally on medium heat.

Mix in the broth juice. Put in the wine and let it boil. Put in thyme, mace, salt, dill and weed and mix them well. Put in shrimp.

Cook till heated throughout. Whisk in cream just prior to serving. Top soup if needed with some slim slices of mushroom and fresh parsley.

Cod With Oregano

Ingredients:

1 tablespoon = fresh oregano (chopped)

1 tablespoon = orange juice

1 tablespoon = olive oil

1 1/2 lbs = cod fish fillets

1 tablespoon = lemon juice

1/2 teaspoon = salt

Directions:

Pre-heat the oven to 450 degrees. In a basin, combine jointly the lemon juice, orange juice, oregano, olive oil and Salt.

Put the fillets on the baking sheet. Cover the fish with the dressing. Bake the cod for 10 minutes. Serve right away.

Ritz Fish

Ingredients:

1/2 cup = butter

4 = fish fillets

32 = Ritz crackers

Directions:

Rinse fish filets and dry them. Place filets in a baking tray. Keep aside. Place Ritz crackers in a baggie and break the crackers to a fine crush.

Put in butter to the Ritz and mix up well. Put the Ritz mixture on the top of all the filets. Cook in the oven at 350 degrees for 25 - 30 minutes.

Check by placing a fork in the fish. The fish should be crunchy and the Ritz crackers should be well browned. Eat instantly.

Lori's Oil Poached Fish

Ingredients:

Olive oil

4 = firm fleshed fish fillets

2 = garlic cloves (minced)

3 tablespoons = parsley

Lemon wedges

Fresh ground pepper

Salt

Directions:

Wash and dry the fish. Transfer sufficient oil in a deep pan. Include the garlic and parsley as well.

Let it fry and add fish into it. Simmer over low heat for almost 14 minutes.

Take away fish. Remove excess oil, if any. Put it on plates. Season it. Dish up with lemons.

Chapter 5 - Desserts

The Ultimate Punch

Ingredients:

1 = package powdered lemonade mix
6 ounce = strawberry Jell-O gelatin
2 liters = ginger ale
1/2 gallon = pineapple juice
2 cups = sugar

Directions:
Combine all ingredients jointly and freeze up in a zip paper bag. Thaw 40 minutes before serving.
Include Ginger Ale and serve up. It will be frosty, but will liquefy as your party goes on.

Chocolate Energy Bars

Ingredients:

11/2 cups = dried dates (pitted)
1 cup = dark chocolate chip (roughly chopped)
11/2 cups = peanuts (unsalted)
1/4 tsp = salt

Directions:

Mix the pitted dates, peanuts and salt in a blender.

Blend 5 to 6 times to crumble the ingredients. Take away the lid and cut up any clumps of dates.

Put back the lid and blend constantly for 1 minute till the ingredients start to clump jointly. When you take away the lid, the ingredients might even now look a little flaky but should grasp together when pushed in your fist.

Drop 1/2 cup of the chocolate on the peanut-date mixture. Put back the lid and blend just 3 to 4 times to incorporate the chocolate.

Shift the mixture to the baking plate and push it tightly down with the palm of your hand or the base of a drinking cup. Dissolve the left over 1/2 cups of chocolate chips in 15-second bursts in the microwave, moving between each burst.

Transfer the melted chocolate on the bars and make use of a spatula to spread it into a smooth layer.

Cover up the bars and keep cold for as a minimum an hour or all night, till the bars are hard and the chocolate is set.

With the bars still in the dish, make use of a sharp knife to slice them into bars. Bars will stay for almost a month refrigerated or for almost a week if unrefrigerated.

Chocolate Strawberry Mousse

Ingredients:

1 = Strawberry
½ Scoop = Chocolate Whey Powder
⅓ Cup = Heavy Whipping Cream
Flakes of = Chocolate
4 Drops = EZ-Sweet
2.5 g = Unsweetened Cocoa

Directions:
Measure the cream into a pot. Put in the sweetener. Also add the strawberry, powder, chocolate flakes and mix for 1-2 minutes or till hard.

Eggnog

Ingredients:
1/4 cup = heavy cream
1/4 cup = egg substitute
1/4 tsp = vanilla extract
1/3 cup = cold water
1 dash = nutmeg

Directions:
Combine everything excluding the nutmeg together. If the water was not cold, cool till cold. You can also alternate a couple of ice cubes for some of the cold water. Dust with nutmeg. Spike with rum and enjoy!

Coffee Cooler

Ingredients:

6 fluid ounces = espresso
2 fluid ounces = cream
1 teaspoon = sugar substitute
1 cup = crushed ice
1 dash = cinnamon

Directions:

Blend all the ingredients in blender till smooth and Enjoy.

Homemade Whipped Cream

Ingredients:

¼ tsp = EZ- Sweetz
200 mL = Heavy Cream
¼ tsp = Vanilla

Directions:

Mix all ingredients and put in ISI Mini Easy Whip Container Charge with N2O cartridge. Mix 3-4 times, if it becomes runny, shake well more. Serve as it is or on top of a food and drink.

Coconut Macaroons

Ingredients:

1 tsp = Vanilla
4 = Egg Whites
4½ tsp = Water

½ tsp = EZ-Sweet

120 g = Unsweetened Coconut

Directions:

Mix egg whites and other liquids. Put in Coconut and mix well. If the mixture is too loose, hit it with the immersion blender to reduce the coconut size and fix the mixture more.

Put on a greased pie pot.

Heat the oven to 375, when you place the macaroons in, decrease the heat to 325.

Cook in the oven for 14 minutes.

Chocolate Hearts

Ingredients:

2 Oz. = Coconut Oil

1 teaspoon = Cocoa Powder

1 Oz. = Cream Cheese

2 Oz. = Almond Butter

½ Oz. = Torani Sugar Free Vanilla Syrup

2 Oz = Dark Chocolate (I Used 85%)

8 Drops = EZ-Sweetz

Directions:

Mix all the stuff but not the almond butter and microwave for 30 seconds. Mix the ingredients, if the chocolate is not completely melted, microwave once again and keep on moving.

Add a base layer into the mold. Then by a spoon place a blob of Almond Butter in the middle. Fill up the mold to the top. Freeze up till the chocolate hardens, as hard press on them out of the mold. Keep in the fridge.

Mint Chocolate Chip Ice Cream

Ingredients:
½ tsp = Liquid Stevia Extract
Several Drops = Peppermint Extract
1 Square = Dark Chocolate
1 Cup = Heavy Cream
½ tsp = Vanilla
½ Cup = Light Cream
Several Drops = Green food coloring

Directions:
Put ice cream bowl in freezer normally 4-12 hours.
Place all ingredients except chocolate in metal dish.
Whip and set back in freezer for 5 minutes.
Setup ice cream maker and put in liquid.
Some minutes before the ice cream is done, put in chocolate shavings.
Put in an air tight box and set back in the freezer.

Almond Cakes

Ingredients:

¾ Cup = Almond Flour
2 = Large Eggs
5 Tbsp = Unsalted Butter
1.5 tsp = Baking Powder

Directions:
Mix the dry ingredients in a basin. Beat the eggs. Melt butter and add to mixture and mix.
Separate mixture equally into 6 portions, put into a Muffin pan. Cook in the oven for almost 12-17 minutes at 350 degrees. Cool on a wire stand.

Almond Bun Pizza

Ingredients:

2 = Eggs
5 Tbsp = Butter
¾ Cup = Almond Meal
122 g (1/2 Cup) = Alfredo sauce
2 oz = Jarhlsberg
½ tsp = Garlic Powder
½ tsp = Oregano
1.5 tsp = Baking Powder
4 oz = Cheddar
1.5 tsp = Splenda
¼ tsp = Thyme

Directions:

Combine the dry ingredients and mix up well.

Ensure that the eggs are warm by placing them in hot water prior to use. Include eggs to dry ingredients.

Melt butter then put in to the mixture.

pray Pam on pizza pan and extend mixture to pizza pan. Cook at 350 degrees for almost 6 minutes.

Add Alfredo sauce to pizza.

Also add cheese to pizza and any other toppings as well.

Broil for almost 2 minutes.

Chapter 6 - Others

Western Scrambled Eggs

Ingredients:

10 = Eggs

225 g = Diced Ham

120 mL = Heavy Cream

113 g = Green Onions

100 mL = Water

8 Oz = Cheddar Cheese

234 g = Diced Tomatoes (drained)

Garlic Powder

Onion Powder

Salt

Pepper

Directions:

Pre-heat the oven to 450 degrees. Beat Eggs, Water, Cream and Spices together. Cover a large cookie sheet with oil and then add eggs. Cook for almost 8 minutes and then add toppings. Cook for 2 more minutes or till the cheese has melted. Cool for 5 minutes or till pan is cool enough to touch. Scramble the mixture and ready to eat.

Brussels Sprout Burgers

Ingredients:

32 oz = Brussels Sprouts (907 g)

36 g = Green Onion

8 oz = Parmesan Cheese

⅓ Cup = Almond Flour

3 = Eggs

11 oz = Goat Cheese

Salt and Pepper (to taste)

Directions:

Rinse Brussels sprouts and cut in a food processor.

Lightly grate the Parmesan and combine with the Brussels sprouts with the almond flour, salt and pepper.

Crush the goat cheese onto the mixture and make use of your hands to mix. Whip three eggs jointly and mix with the mixture.

Patty out 4 oz burgers! Warm oil in a skillet! Fry the burgers for 2.5 minutes per side till crunchy.

Chorizo Breakfast Casserole

Ingredients:

12 = eggs

110 g = Onion (1 small)

16 Oz = Ground Chorizo

180 g = Heavy Cream (12 Tbsp)

366 g = Spinach

8 Oz = Cheddar

9 Oz = Cherry Tomatoes

145 g = Green Pepper (1 small)
Garlic Powder, Onion Powder, Salt, and Pepper (to taste)

Directions:
Bake the spinach in the microwave. Crush or chop the chorizo and fry in a skillet till browned. Put completed chorizo in a large basin.

Finely slice 1 onion and 1 pepper and cook in the same skillet, as completed put in the large basin. At the same time when the spinach is done, put in the basin as well. Beat together the eggs, cream and spices.

Put in the cheese to the basin and mix, and then put in the egg mixture and mix. Shift to a greased dish. Include cherry tomatoes. Cook at 350 degrees for nearly 50 minutes.

Bacon Hash

Ingredients:
6 Slices = Bacon
4 = Eggs
1 = Small Pepper
Several slices = Jalapenos
1 = Small Onion

Directions:
Cut the pepper and onions into slim strips.

Cut up the jalapeno slices as tiny as possible. Sauté the vegetables in a pan! Take away when the veggies are transparent and browning.

Chop the bacon in a blender till it cracks into chunks, you don't need to overdo it and finish up with a paste.

Combine all the ingredients collectively.

Prepare the hash till the bacon is getting close to crisp.

Arrange on a platter and top with a fried egg!

Deep Fried Eggs

Ingredients:

2 =Eggs

3 Slices = Bacon

Directions:

Warm some oil in a fryer to 375 degrees. Cook bacon. Put two eggs into a bowl. Quickly fall the egg into the center of the fryer, do not fall them in, and try to break them in near the surface, but be alert since the oil is hot.

By two spatulas, corral the egg into a ball, it may stay in one piece or it may choose to go all over the place. Fry till it stops bubbling, 3-4 minutes Let drain on some paper towels!

Baked Eggs

Ingredients:

4 = Slices Bacon
1 = Small Onion
1 Oz = Cheddar
4 = Eggs
Salt and Pepper (to taste)

Directions:
Stir fry four slices of bacon. Cut an onion in half and sauté. In a ramekin, put onion and bacon.
Break two eggs into each pot; be sure to not crack yolk. Put in salt and pepper. Also add cheddar cheese. Cook in the oven at 350 degrees for 20 minutes or till eggs have set!

Deviled Egg Chicks

Ingredients:
1 Tbsp = Dijon Mustard
10 = Eggs
Hot Sauce
4 Tbsp = Mayo
Olive Slivers
Carrot Slivers

Directions:
Put the eggs in a skillet filled with water and boil. When boiling, keep on boiling for 15 minutes. Shock the eggs with cold water, and then peel off. Cut in half and split out the egg yolks.

In a dish, mix the egg yolks, mayo, mustard and hot sauce. Stir till smooth. Trim the bottoms off of half the egg halves and the center of the remaining.

Put in the yolk mixture onto the bottoms, ensuring that to include more to the front side. Finish with all of the eggs and put a carrot and two olive slices for the nose and eyes.

Atkins Lightly Spicy Turnip Fries

Ingredients:
4 = turnips (trimmed and peeled)
1/2 teaspoon = chili powder
2 tablespoons = olive oil
1 teaspoon = kosher salt

Directions:
Pre-heat the oven to 425 °F. Slice turnips into sticks. Put on a roll pan. Sprinkle with oil, salt and chili powder.

Flip with hands to cover. Spread in a one layer. Bake fries for 30 minutes, rotating during cooking time for browning. Dish up right away.

Almond Buns

Ingredients:
2 Large = Eggs
¾ Cup = Almond Flour
1.5 tsp = Baking Powder

5 Tbsp = Unsalted Butter

Directions:
Mix the dry ingredients in a basin. Beat in the eggs.
Melt butter and add to mixture and mix. Divide mixture evenly into 6 parts, put into a Muffin. Cook in the oven for 12-17 minutes at 350 degrees. Cool on a wire stand.

Taco Salad

Ingredients:
32 oz = Ground Pork
6 tsp = Taco Seasoning
9 oz = Cheddar Cheese, shredded
12 Tbsp = Salsa
12 Tbsp = Sour Cream
6 = Romaine Leafs
Cayenne Pepper

Directions:
Brown the pork in a pot. When the meat is browned, put in taco seasoning and any extra spices. Fry until the taco seasoning is incorporated. Allow it cool, and then divide into 6 boxes. Put in cheese to each box. Put in sour cream and salsa to a basin and cover it. Include Romaine Lettuce to box.

Tomato-Mozzarella Stacks

Ingredients:
3 1/2 tbsps = salad dressing
8 slices = fresh tomatoes 4 slices fresh mozzarella

Directions:
Cut tomatoes and fresh mozzarella into slices almost the same thickness and diameter. Compose stacks with a piece of tomato, a piece of fresh mozzarella, and one more piece of tomato, and then pour salad Dressing over every stack.

Pita Pizza

Ingredients:
2 Oz = Cheddar Cheese
1 Oz = Roasted Red Peppers
1 = Low Carb Pita
14 = slices Pepperoni
½ Cup = Tomato Basil Marinara Sauce

Directions:
Divide the low carb pita in half and put on a foil lined sheet.
Grease with some olive oil and toast for 1-2 minutes at 450 degrees to make it crunchy.
Put the sauce over the pita bread.
Cover with cheese as well as with toppings.
Cook for an extra 5 minutes in order to melt the cheese.

Chicken Broccoli Soup

Ingredients:
12 oz = Cheddar Cheese, Shredded
1 Can = Chicken Broth
8 = Chicken Thighs
1.5 cups = Heavy Cream
4 Slices = Bacon
780 g = Broccoli
Salt, pepper, garlic powder and onion powder (To Taste)

Directions:
Pre-heat oven to 350 degrees! Put chicken thighs in saucepan with a lid, add spices, and also water. Cook chicken for almost 2 hours.
When chicken is cooking, sauté 4 slices of bacon. Fry Broccoli as well in bacon grease, and mash the broccoli as much as possible with spatula. As chicken is ready and cooled, put into container.
Put in broccoli and bacon, combine over medium heat. Include cheese, heavy cream and broth. Heat till thickened.

Roasted Duck

Ingredients:

1 = Duck

Directions:
Wash the duck and eliminate surplus fat and any related extras like the liver, heart, neck, etc. Bind the legs jointly.
Cook at 300 degrees for almost 3 hours, rotating and pushing with a knife every 30 minutes, you should push from side to side the skin but not penetrating the meat. Perhaps 25 or so pushes and you should see fat discharge out of the pokes. Divide into four parts and serve!

Bourbon Glazed Ham

Ingredients:
1 tsp. = Champagne Vinegar
8-12 Lb = Bone-in Ham Shank
2 Oz. = Bourbon
1¼ Cup = Splenda
1 tsp. = Ground Mustard
Cloves

Directions:
Cut fat and crisscross the ham. Put in a roasting pan and add an inch of water and cook for an hour at 325 degrees covered.
Arrange glaze by mixing all the glaze ingredients excluding the cloves.
After an hour, eliminate most of the water.

Add the glaze to the ham and put the cloves in the crisscross areas. Cook for further an hour open.
Enjoy!

Bacon Cheddar Cauliflower Soup

Ingredients:
4 = Slices Bacon
12 Oz. = Aged Cheddar
1 = Cauliflower Head
¼ Cup = Heavy Cream
2 Tbsp = Olive Oil
3 Cups = Chicken Broth
1 = Medium Onion
1 tsp = Ground Thyme
1 Tbsp = Minced Garlic
1 Oz = Parmesan Cheese

Directions:
Chop up the cauliflower, put it on a foil lined sheet, and sprinkle with olive oil.
Add Salt and pepper the cauliflower and bacon and bake at 375 degrees for 35 minutes. Cook the bacon till crunchy; if possible make use of a large pan that can fit the soup.
Cut up a medium onion and sauté it in the bacon grease.
Just the once the onion is ended, put in the garlic and thyme and cook for 30 seconds.

Put in the Chicken Broth and cauliflower, then cook covered for nearly 20 minutes.

When the cauliflower is cooking, grate some aged cheddar. Using a blender, blend the cauliflower.

Put in the cheese and mix together more.

Put in the bacon and cream and combine together with a spoon.

Keto Dip

Ingredients:
8 Oz = Sour Cream
20 Oz = Guacamole
4 Oz = Mayonnaise
4 Oz = Cream cheese
4 Oz = Green Onions, Diced
2 Tablespoons = Taco Seasoning
16 Oz = Salsa
10 Oz = Cheddar Cheese, Shredded

Directions:
Begin by mixing the mayo, cream cheese, sour cream and seasoning. Mix up till soft. Cut up the green onions as well.

Take a medium sized casserole dish; begin by spreading out the guacamole on the base. Then cautiously spread the sour cream mixture on top of the guacamole.

Now put the salsa on the sour cream mixture. Include the cheese. Finish with green onions.

This is good if you allow it sit in the refrigerator for at least 1 hour and up to 24 for the flavors to mix together.

Fried Broccoli

Ingredients:
1 Bunch = Broccoli
2 Oz = Bleu Cheese Dressing
1 tsp = Red Hot

Directions:
Break the florets from the broccoli. Deep fry till golden brown and crunchy. When the broccoli is frying, mix the bleu cheese and red hot. Serve with the sauce!

Spinach Crap

Ingredients:
½ = Onion Soup Packet
30 Oz = Frozen Spinach
2 Cups = Sour Cream
4 Oz = Colby Jack Cheese (shredded)
4 Oz = Cheddar Cheese (shredded)

Directions:
Thaw the spinach in the microwave and dry it. Put in the cheese, sour cream, and half of an onion soup packet. Combine and add to a greased casserole dish. Drop extra cheese on top. Bake for 35 minutes at 375 degrees. Enjoy!

Spicy Fried Brussels Sprouts

Ingredients:
1 lb 8 oz = Brussels sprouts
1 tsp = Lime Juice
2 Oz = Mayo
0.5 Oz = Srirachi

Directions:
Rinse and then divide into four parts the Brussels sprouts. Cook them in batches; ensure that not to overload the fryer. Cook for 6 minutes or till golden brown. Combine the liquid ingredients, then mix with the Brussels sprouts and enjoy!

Creamy Cheesy Spinach

Ingredients:
255 g = Spinach
58 g = Cheddar Cheese (shredded)
4 Tbsp = Cream Cheese

Directions:
Soften spinach on medium heat. Heat till the spinach is soft and the juices are reduced. Put in cream cheese, combine till incorporated. Put in cheese, combine till incorporated.

Mashed Cauliflower

Ingredients:

1 Head = Cauliflower
5 Slices = Bacon
2 Oz. = Cream Cheese
2½ Oz. = Monterey Jack Cheese
2½ Oz. = Cheddar Cheese
Salt and Pepper to taste

Directions:

Cook the bacon and then crush. Rinse and cut up the cauliflower. Let some water to a boil and then include the cauliflower and boil for further 9 minutes.

As the cauliflower is boiling, dice the cheeses. Strain the cauliflower. Crush the cauliflower, and then put in the cream cheese and mash.

Add salt and pepper. Mix in the cheese and bacon. Shift to a baking plate and bake for 10 minutes at 350 degrees.

Valentine's Day Eggs For Two – Phase 1

Serves 2

Ingredients:

4 eggs

2 c. fresh, chopped spinach

3 tsp. heavy cream

1 Tbsp. butter

2 oz. goat cheese

Salt & pepper to taste

1. Preheat oven to 325 degrees.
2. Beat eggs and cream until fully combined. Mix in chopped spinach. Add salt and pepper to taste.
3. Coat two ramekins with butter, then spoon mixture in. Bake for 10 minutes.
4. Sprinkle on cheese, then bake for 3 more minutes.
5. Serve warm.

Valentine's Day Crab Cakes – Phase 1

Serves 4

Ingredients:

12oz. crabmeat

2 eggs

1/4 c. diced celery

1/4 c. diced green onion

1/4 c. diced red pepper

2 Tbsp. parmesan

1 Tbsp. extra virgin olive oil

1. Combine everything but oil in a bowl. Press into four patties and put on line cookie sheet in the refrigerator for at least half an hour.

2. Heat large skillet on medium heat. Add olive oil.

3. Gently place patties into oil spaced far enough that they do not touch. Cook until browned, then flip and cook an additional 3 minutes.

4. Serve immediately with garlic butter sauce or freeze for up to two weeks.

Valentine's Day Heart-Y Pot Pies – Phase 3

Serves 8

Ingredients:

3 eggs

1/8 tsp. Cream of Tartar

3 oz. cream cheese

1 c. cooked lean ground turkey

1 c. heavy cream

1/4 c. chopped broccoli

1 chopped carrot

2 Tbsp. butter

1/4 c. parmesan

1/2 c. mozzarella

1. Preheat oven to 350 degrees.
2. Separate eggs into two bowls.
3. To the whites, add Cream of Tartar, and beat until stiff peaks form.
4. To the yolks, add cream cheese and blend until smooth.
5. Slowly fold white mixture in with yolk mixture until just combined.
6. Grease four small heart-shaped pans. Separate equal parts of mixture to each, pressing until it forms to sides. Bake for 30 minutes.
7. While crusts bake, mix cooked turkey, heavy cream, mozzarella, broccoli, and carrot in a medium pot. Cook over medium heat until carrots start to tenderize.
8. When crusts come out of the oven, add equal parts of filling to each. Add parmesan and mozzarella to top, and bake again for 10 minutes until cheese is bubbly. Serve hot.

Valentine's Day Chococado Smoothies – Phase 2

Serves 2

Ingredients:
1 avocado, mashed
2 Tbsp. unsweetened cocoa powder
1/2 c. heavy cream
2 tsp. sweetener

1/2 c. water

1 c. ice

1. Combine all ingredients in a blender and pulse until fully combined.

2. Serve in a pretty glass with a sprig of mint on top for garnish.

St. Patrick's Day Green Frittata – Phase 1

Serves 2

Ingredients:

4 eggs

6 stalks of asparagus, quartered

1/2 c. bell pepper, diced

2 sprigs rosemary

2 oz. goat cheese

1 Tbsp. butter

1. Preheat oven to 400 degrees. Grease the bottom and sides of a small cake pan.

2. In a bowl, combine goat cheese and eggs. Whisk until combined.

3. Arrange asparagus and bell pepper on the bottom of the pan. Pour cheese and egg mixture on top. Sprinkle rosemary on top.

4. Bake 14 – 17 minutes, or until the center is firm and cheese starts to brown. Serve warm.

St. Patrick's Corned Beef And Cabbage Hash – Phase 2

Serves 2

Ingredients:

16 oz. corned beef

2 c. cooked turnips

1/2 c. plain Greek yogurt

1/2 c. onions, chopped

2 Tbsp. olive oil

1 c. fresh cabbage, chopped

1. Heat large skillet over medium-low heat.

2. Combine beef, turnips, yogurt, and onions in a large bowl.

3. Drizzle olive oil to skillet and let warm 1 minute. Add contents of bowl to skillet and cook, without stirring, for 8 – 12 minutes.

4. Flip hash and cook for another 8 minutes.

5. Add cabbage and steam, covered, for 1 minute.

6. Serve immediately.

St. Paddy's Day Dinner Salad – Phase 1

Serves 8

Ingredients:

4 Tbsp. extra virgin olive oil

8 boneless skinless chicken breasts

3 c. romaine

1 c. arugula

1 c. fresh broccoli

1 green bell pepper

2 stalks celery

2 avocados

1 c. alfalfa sprouts

3 Tbsp. lemon juice

Salt and pepper to taste

1. Heat oven to 400 degrees. Grease a baking pan with 1 Tbsp. of olive oil, season chicken breasts, and arrange them in a single layer on the pan.
2. Bake for 25 – 30 minutes uncovered or until chicken is no longer pink in the center.
3. Chop lettuce, arugula, broccoli, bell pepper, celery, and avocados.
4. Combine chopped ingredients in a large serving bowl with sprouts, oil, and lemon juice. Toss well.
5. When the chicken is cooked, slice it into strips and place even amounts on each of the 8 individual salads. Serve immediately.

St. Patrick's Green Smoothie – Phase 4

Serves 5

Ingredients:

2 c. coconut milk

1/3 c. coconut oil

5 individual plain low-carb shake mixes

5 inches vanilla beans, scraped

3 small bananas

2 c. spinach

3 c. ice

1. Combine all ingredients in a blender until well combined.
2. Serve immediately.

Mardi Gras Faux Beignets – Phase 4

Serves 4

Ingredients:

2 eggs

1/3 c. room temperature water

2 Tbsp. warm butter

2 Tbsp. almond flour

1 Tbsp. sweetener

1/4 tsp. baking powder

4 Tbsp. butter

1/2 c. powdered sweetener

Metal cookie cutter

1. Mix water and warm butter until combined in one bowl.
2. Mix flour, 1 Tbsp. sweetener, and baking powder in another.
3. Whisk dry mixture into wet mixture until combined and there are no remaining lumps.
4. Heat a small skillet over medium-high heat.
5. Add 1 Tbsp. butter to skillet and allow to just melt.
6. Pour one quarter of batter into cookie cutter in center of skillet and allow to cook on one side for about one minute. Cover skillet for an additional minute of cooking.

7. Uncover, remove cookie cutter, and flip beignet to cook on the other side for 2 more minutes.

8. Repeat steps 5 – 7 until all beignets are made. Dust warm faux beignets with powdered sweetener and serve immediately.

Mardi Gras Muffalettas – Phase 4

Serves 2

Ingredients:
2 thin slices of Swiss cheese
4 thin slices of ham
4 thin slices of salami
4 Tbsp. olive salad
4 slices low-carb bread, like Trader Joe's Sprouted (4 net carbs)

1. Toast bread lightly. Spread 1 Tbsp. olive salad on each piece of bread.
2. Place 1 slice of Swiss, 2 slices of ham, and 2 slices of salami on each sandwich.
3. Put it together and serve it with kale chips or a side salad.

Mardi Gras Seafood Gumbo – Phase 2

Serves 10

Ingredients:

4 c. warm vegetable broth

4 c. warm water

8 Tbsp. almond flour

8 Tbsp. extra virgin olive oil

2 c. crabmeat

2 c. cleaned shrimp

10 oz. chopped okra

1/2 c. chopped scallions

1/2 c. diced green bell peppers

1/2 c. diced celery

1 head of cauliflower

1. Heat a large pot over medium-high heat. Add half of olive oil, scallions, celery, and bell peppers. Sautee until they glisten and soften.

2. Add the rest of the olive oil, then add the flour slowly, mixing constantly until the roux starts to turn reddish brown. DO NOT ALLOW THE ROUX TO BURN.

3. Take the pot off the burner. Add brother and water slowly, stirring continuously until it is well combined. (At this stage, add 1 cup at a time of broth, then water, until you reach the consistency you want.)

4. Add cleaned shrimp, crabmeat, and okra. Bring to a boil, then turn down heat to simmer. Cook for about an hour and a half.

5. While gumbo is cooking, preheat oven to 425 degrees. Then roughly chop raw cauliflower and drop into a food processor. Process until evenly chopped.

6. Spread cauliflower out in a thin, even layer on a nonstick cookie sheet. Bake for 8 minutes, flip, then bake for 7 more minutes.

7. Spoon "rice" out into bowls, then add a serving of gumbo on top. Serve immediately with crackers and hot sauce.

Mardi Gras King Cake Minis – Phase 3

Serves 4

Ingredients:

CAKE

3 eggs

1/8 tsp. Cream of Tartar

3 oz. softened cream cheese

1 tsp. baking powder

2 Tbsp. sugar free vanilla syrup

ICING

1 oz. cream cheese

3 Tbsp. butter

2 Tbsp. heavy cream

1 vanilla bean

1 Tbsp. sugar free vanilla syrup

6 drops liquid sweetener

Red, yellow, and green food dye

SUGAR TOPPING

1 tsp. powdered sweetener

1. Preheat oven to 300 degrees.
2. In a small bowl, whip together egg whites and Cream of Tartar.
3. In a medium-sized bowl, combine egg yolks, softened cream cheese, baking powder, and vanilla syrup.

4. Fold white mixture with yolk mixture until just combined.
5. Pour batter into small cake pans, and bake for 30 minutes.
6. Blend cream cheese, butter, and heavy cream in another bowl until combined.
7. Scrape in vanilla, then add vanilla syrup and liquid sweetener.
8. Separate icing into three small bowls. Add red food coloring to one, yellow to another, and green to the last and mix until the color is consistent.
9. Allow cakes to cool completely, then coat each cake with the separate colors of icing and sprinkle with sweetener for texture.

Easter Egg Muffins – Phase 1

Serves 12

Ingredients:

15 eggs
1 green bell pepper
2 Tbsp. diced green onions
1 clove of garlic, minced
1 c. low-fat shredded cheddar

1. Preheat oven to 375 degrees and line muffin tin with paper liners.
2. In a large bowl, whisk eggs until frothy. Add in bell pepper, onions, and garlic.
3. Scoop mixture until muffin liners until about 2/3 full to allow room to rise.
4. Bake muffins for about 30 minutes or until they are slightly

browned on top.

5. Serve warm or refrigerate for up to one week.

Easter Cauli-Egg Salad – Phase 2

Serves 10

Ingredients:

2 c. cauliflower

3 hard-boiled eggs, chopped

1/4 c. light sour cream

1/4 c. plain Greek yogurt

1 tsp. mustard

1/4 c. green onions, diced

1. Chop cauliflower into one inch cubes and steam for about five minutes. Remove from heat and allow to cool.

2. Add chopped eggs and onion to cauliflower, then mix in sour cream, yogurt, and mustard.

3. Chill in refrigerator for 20 minutes before serving. Sprinkle with paprika or bacon bits, or garnish with dill for a pop of color.

Easter Roasted Brisket – Phase 3

Servings vary based on size of brisket

Ingredients:

Beef brisket point half

3 stalks of celery, quartered

3 carrots, quartered

1 white onion, quartered
2 garlic cloves, minced
3 Tbsp. balsamic vinegar
Salt and black pepper
Water to cover

1. Chop vegetables and place them on the bottom of your crockpot. Add balsamic vinegar.
2. Trim layer of fat from the surface using a sharp knife. Chop the brisket in half if necessary to fit into the crockpot, and place it on top of the vegetables.
3. Season entire contents with salt and black pepper to taste.
4. Cover with water and cook on low for 12 hours or high for 6 hours.
5. Slice and serve with the cooked vegetables as a side. Cover it all with the cooking liquid as a sauce.

Easter Carrot Cottontails – Phase 3

Serves 12
Ingredients:
3 eggs
1 c. vegetable oil
1-1/2 c. sweetener
1 tsp. baking soda
1 tsp. cinnamon
1 vanilla bean
1-1/2 c. almond flour

1/2 c. flax seed meal

3 c. shredded carrots

Bunny-shaped cookie cutter

1. Preheat oven to 350 degrees.
2. In a large bowl, mix eggs, oil, and sweetener.
3. Add the rest of the ingredients and stir until well combined.
4. Pour batter into a 9" x 13" nonstick pan, and bake until a knife inserted in the center comes out clean (about half an hour).
5. Let cool and cut with bunny-shaped cookie cutter into servings.
6. Serve alone or with a light coating of cream cheese.

Fourth Of July Cheesy Apple Strudel – Phase 4

Serves 4

Ingredients:

2 medium apples

4 dates, pitted

1 c. quinoa

2 c. water

1 tsp. apple pie spice

3 tsp. sweetener

1. Rinse and drain quinoa.
2. Peel and core apples. Dice apples and dates into small pies.

3. In a medium sauce pan, combine water, quinoa, apples, and dates. Bring to a boil, then simmer for about 15 minutes.

4. Stir in apple pie spice and sweetener until well combined.
5. Serve hot. Add a dollop of heavy cream or plain yogurt for a little extra burst of flavor.

Fourth Of July Cbt Snacks – Phase 1

Serves 10

Ingredients:
20 slices thick-cut bacon
4 large tomatoes
20 oz. goat cheese

1. Cut slices of bacon in half and weave together into 10 individual grids on two nonstick baking sheets using two (whole) pieces per grid.
2. Bake at 400 degrees (don't preheat!) for 17 to 20 minutes.
3. While the bacon is in the oven, cut tomatoes into thick inch slices. Gently slice the goat cheese into thin slices.
4. Take bacon out of oven and allow to cool, then top evenly with tomato slices and goat cheese. Serve immediately.

Fourth Of July Spicy Chicken Wraps – Phase 4

Serves 6

Ingredients:
2 tsp. salt

2 tsp. pepper

3 tsp. oregano

4 tsp. parsley

2 tsp. cayenne pepper

2 Tbsp. butter

24 boneless chicken pieces

6 large cabbage leaves

12 Tbsp. ranch dressing

1. Preheat oven to 350 degrees. Line a baking sheet with foil and place a cooking rack on top.
2. In a pie tin, mix salt, pepper, and spices until combined.
3. In a separate, small bowl, melt the butter until liquefied.
4. Dip chicken pieces in butter, then roll in spice mix. Put each piece on the rack until full.
5. Bake for about an hour, until the outside is crispy and the inside is no longer pink.
6. Wrap chicken in cabbage leaves and drizzle with ranch dressing. Serve hot.

Fourth Of July Red, White, And Berries – Phase 3

Serves 4

Ingredients:

1/2 c. fresh blackberries

1/2 c. fresh strawberries

1/2 c. fresh raspberries

1/2 c. fresh blueberries
1/2 c. ricotta cheese
1/2 c. cottage cheese
2 tsp. sweetener
1/4 c. shaved raw almonds

1. In a large bowl, combine cheeses and sweetener. Whisk until well creamed.
2. Gently fold in berries until combined. Refrigerate for half an hour.
3. Spoon equal amounts of cheese and berry mix into serving bowls. Top with shaved almonds and serve immediately.

Memorial/Veterans Day Biscuits & Gravy – Phase 4

Serves 9

Ingredients:
BISCUITS
1-1/4 c. almond flour
2 Tbsp. cold butter
1 tsp. baking powder
3 egg whites
GRAVY
2 c. water
2 chicken bouillon cubes
2 Tbsp. room temperature butter
2 Tbsp. corn starch

1. Preheat oven to 375 degrees. Grease muffin tin.
2. In a small bowl, whisk egg whites.
3. In a separate, medium mixing bowl, combine dry biscuit ingredients, then cut in cold butter.
4. Combine egg whites with flour mixture.
5. Spoon biscuit batter into muffin tins about 2/3 full.
6. Bake for 12 – 14 minutes or until golden brown on top.
7. While biscuits are baking, combine water, bouillon cubes, and room temperature butter in a medium sauce pan. Bring to a boil.
8. Whisk in corn starch slowly, and stir continuously for 2 minutes.
9. Split biscuits in half, two per plate, and cover with equal amounts of gravy. Serve warm.

Memorial/Veterans Day Game Hens - Phase 3

Serves 4

Ingredients:
4 Cornish game hens
1/3 c. butter
1/3 c. chopped onions
1 c. chopped celery
1 c. chopped carrots
1 tsp. parsley
1 tsp. rosemary
Salt and pepper to taste

1. Preheat oven to 375 degrees. Tie drumsticks of hens together.
2. Heat butter, onions, celery, parsley, and rosemary to sauce pan. Heat for 2 – 3 minutes.
3. Spread carrots in a single layer in the bottom of a tall-sided roasting pan. Place hens, breast side up, into pan on top of carrots. Spoon butter mixture over it all.
4. Cover pan with foil and bake, basting every 20 minutes with butter mixture, for 80 minutes, or until meat thermometer reads 180 degrees.
5. Serve alone, over cauliflower rice, or with low-carb bread.

Memorial/Veterans Day No-Tortilla Fajitas – Phase 1

Serves 4

Ingredients:
1 lb. skirt steak
3 Tbsp. butter
Juice of 3 limes
2 cloves garlic, minced
2 tsp. chili powder
3 tsp. black pepper
2 tsp. cumin
2 tsp. salt
1 onion, cut into strips
1 each yellow, red, and green bell pepper, cut into strips

1 c. cabbage, cut into strips

1. Allow steak to come to room temperature.
2. Heat grill pan to high heat before adding 1 Tbsp. of butter.
3. Grill skirt steak about 3 minutes.
4. Add remaining butter, lime juice, garlic, and spices to glass mixing bowl. Heat briefly in microwave until butter is melted.
5. Flip and brush steak with part of butter mixture. Place onions, bell pepper, and cabbage into bowl and toss with butter mixture.
6. Remove steak from grill, and place buttered vegetables onto grill. Allow to cook for only 30 seconds.
7. Chop steak into strips and lay out on plates. Top with vegetables and serve hot alone or with guacamole.

Memorial/Veterans Day Cheesecake Flags – Phase 3

Serves 16

Ingredients:

CRUST
1 c. finely chopped almonds
1 Tbsp. sweetener
4 Tbsp. warm butter
FILLING
40 oz. softened cream cheese
1 c. sweetener

3 eggs
1/2 c. plain Greek yogurt
1 Tbsp. lemon juice
1 vanilla bean

TOPPING

1/2 c. heavy cream
2 tsp. sweetener
1/4 c. any red berries
1/4 c. blueberries

1. Mix together crust ingredients and press into the bottom of a nonstick cookie sheet in an even layer. Refrigerate for 1 hour.

2. Preheat oven to 325 degrees.

3. In a medium mixing bowl, whisk cream cheese and sweetener until well combined. Add eggs and continue to mix until blended. Add yogurt, lemon juice, and vanilla bean scrapings and whisk until well blended.

4. Smooth cream cheese mixture onto cooled crust in an even layer. Bake about 1 hour, or until well set. Cool for 20 minutes, then refrigerator for an additional hour.

5. While cheesecake base cools, beat heavy cream and sweetener until it forms into stiff peaks. Layer whipped topping over cheesecake layer, then cut into 16 individual rectangular portions.

6. Arrange berries into flag shapes and serve immediately.

Halloween Spookyface Fruits – Phase 4

Serves 10

Ingredients:
5 clementines
5 small peaches

1. Wash clementines and peaches well.
2. With a paring knife, cut Jack-o-Lantern faces into fronts of fruits.
3. Serve immediately.

Halloween Itsy Bitsy Spiders – Phase 1

Serves 2

Ingredients:
1/2 c. button mushrooms
1/2 c. alfalfa sprouts
2 oz. shredded mozzarella

1. Wash mushrooms and sprouts well, then pat dry.
2. Heat a large nonstick skillet on low. Arrange mozzarella into two web patterns and allow to cook on one side, then remove from heat.
3. With a fine-tip toothpick, press ends of four sprouts into mushrooms on each side to make the spiders.

4. Arrange spiders on webs and serve.

Halloween Spiced Apple Chicken – Phase 3

Serves 4

Ingredients:
4 boneless skinless chicken breasts
1 Tbsp. lemon juice
1/2 tsp. apple pie spice
2 medium apples
3 Tbsp. butter
1 c. chicken broth
Salt and pepper to taste

1. Salt and pepper chicken breasts and cut into slices.
2. In a small bowl, combine lemon juice and spice. Peel and dice apples, then toss them in lemon juice mixture.
3. Heat butter in a medium skillet over medium-high heat. Add chicken and apples and cook, stirring infrequently, for 5 – 6 minutes.
4. Add broth to skillet and cook for another 3 minutes until a thin gravy starts to form. Serve immediately.

Halloween Goblin Balls – Phase 4

Serves 6

Ingredients:
10 dates, pitted

1/2 c. cherries, stemmed and pitted
1/2 c. shredded coconut

1. Spread coconut out on a nonstick cookie sheet.
2. In food processor, combine dates and cherries. Spoon out with a tablespoon and roll into balls.
3. Roll balls in coconut until covered and leave on cookie sheet.
4. Refrigerate for at least half an hour. Serve chilled.

Thanksgiving Flax Muffin – Phase 2

Serves 2

Ingredients:
2 large eggs
4 Tbsp. flax meal
3 tsp. sweetener
2 tsp. heavy cream
1/2 tsp. baking powder

1. Beat eggs in a small bowl with wire whisk. Slowly add in each additional ingredient, stirring continuously.
2. Pour mixture equally into two coffee mugs, and microwave separately on high for 3 minutes.
3. Serve warm with a little butter and warm, unflavored almond or soy milk.

Thanksgiving Smoky Green Beans – Phase 4

Serves 4

Ingredients:
2 strips bacon, diced
2 Tbsp. green onions, chopped
1 lb. fresh green beans
1/2 c. water
1 Tbsp. lemon juice
Salt and pepper to taste

1. In a large skillet, cook bacon on medium heat until crispy. Remove bacon bits from skillet and drain on paper towels.
2. Add water, onions, and beans to skillet and cook about 3 seconds or until colors brighten and beans are tender.
3. Arrange beans and onions in equal portions on plates, sprinkle with bacon, spritz with lemon juice, and season to taste.

Thanksgiving Stuffed Turkey Omelets – Phase 1

Serves 6

Ingredients:
3 lb. turkey breast half, bone-in
4 Tbsp. butter
1/2 tsp. parsley
1/2 tsp. sage
1/2 tsp. thyme

1/2 tsp. basil
1/2 tsp. onion powder
1/2 tsp. garlic powder
12 egg whites
2/3 c. unsweetened soy milk
Salt and pepper to taste
6 oz. cheddar

1. Combine turkey, 2 Tbsp. butter, and spices in a slow cooker. Cook 5 hours on high or 9 hours on low.
2. Shred turkey breast into a medium bowl and set aside.
3. Heat butter in a large skillet over medium heat.
4. Whisk egg whites and milk with salt and pepper. Pour a thin layer of egg white mixture into skillet.
5. Cook on one side until firm, then flip. Add shredded turkey and cheese.
6. Remove from heat when cheese starts to melt. Plate and serve warm alone or with fresh cranberry* salsa.

* Will elevate phase from 1 to 2.

Thanksgiving Pumpkin Yogurt – Phase 3

Serves 4

Ingredients:
2 c. pureed pumpkin
2 c. plain Greek yogurt

4 tsp. sweetener

8 Tbsp. crushed pecans

1. In a medium mixing bowl, combine pumpkin, yogurt, and sweetener. Whip mixture until it takes on a mousse-like texture.
2. Spoon mixture into serving bowls. Top with pecans and serve.

Christmas Dreamy Sweet Potatoes – Phase 3

Serves 2

Ingredients:

1 medium sweet potato

1 c. shredded coconut

6 dates, pitted

1 c. cottage cheese

2 tsp. sweetener

1. Prick sweet potato several times with fork, then place on a microwave-safe plate. Cook for 9 minutes on high.
2. Dice dates into small pieces.
3. Cut sweet potato into halves, mash, and place into serving bowls.
4. Spoon cottage cheese onto sweet potato. Add coconut and dates. Sprinkle entire dessert with sweetener and serve immediately.

Christmas Festive Coleslaw – Phase 1

Serves 6

Ingredients:
1/2 head of green cabbage
2 red bell peppers
1/4 c. lemon juice
1/4 c. extra virgin olive oil
2 Tbsp. liquid sweetener

1. Thinly chop cabbage and bell peppers into strips.
2. In a medium serving bowl, mix lemon juice, olive oil, and sweetener.
3. Toss cabbage and bell peppers in juice mix.
4. Serve immediately for a fresh salad taste, or refrigerate overnight if you want a more pickled flavor.

Christmas Apple-Stuffed Pork – Phase 3

Serves 4

Ingredients:
1 medium sweet apple
2 Tbsp. extra virgin olive oil
1 lb. pork tenderloin
1/2 c. apple cider vinegar
1-1/3 c. water
2 tsp. cornstarch

1. Preheat oven to 450 degrees.
2. Butterfly the tenderloin and pound to 1/4-inch thickness. Set aside.
3. Peel, core, and chop apple into 1/2-inch cubes.
4. Heat half the oil in large skillet over medium heat. Add apple and sauté about 2 minutes, then remove from skillet.
5. Evenly distribute warm apples inside tenderloin, then roll meat up to seal in the filling. Tie with kitchen string to keep tenderloin closed.
6. Place tenderloin in skillet and brown on all sides, then transfer it to a roasting pan.
7. Whisk vinegar, water, and cornstarch together and pour over tenderloin.
7. Bake for 15 – 20 minutes, or until meat thermometer shows 145 degrees. Serve hot.

Christmas Almond Biscotti – Phase 4

Serves 10

Ingredients:

2 Tbsp. almonds, ground
3-1/2 Tbsp. soy flour
1/2 tsp. salt
1/2 tsp. baking powder

1/2 tsp. ground cinnamon
1/2 tsp. xanthan gum
3 Tbsp. vegetable oil
2 tsp. sweetener
2 eggs
1 vanilla bean
2 Tbsp. almonds, chopped

1. Preheat oven to 325 degrees. Grease a large cookie sheet.
2. In a small mixing bowl, combine ground almonds, flour, salt, baking powder, cinnamon, and xanthan gum.
3. In another bowl, whisk oil, sweetener, eggs, and vanilla bean scrapings. Slowly mix in dry ingredients and chopped almonds.
4. Separate into 2" x 1" loaves and place far apart on the cookie sheet. Bake for 35 – 45 minutes.
5. Remove from heat and reduce temperature to 200 degrees. Slice loaves into 10 – 12 pieces and place the slices back on the cookie sheet with flat sides down.
6. Bake slices for 20 minutes, flipping halfway through.
7. Serve warm or freeze for up to two weeks.

Part 2

Atkins Breakfast Recipes

All Purpose Low-Carb Baking Mix

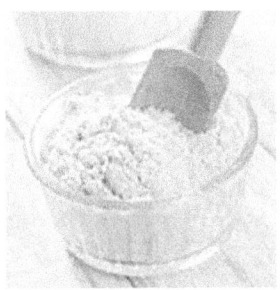

Servings: 9 | **Prep**: 5 mins | **Style:** American

Ingredients
- 1/4 cup Wheat Bran (Crude)
- 1 1/8 cups Whole Grain Soy Flour
- 2/3 cup Vanilla Whey Protein
- 1/4 cup Organic 100% Whole Ground Golden Flaxseed Meal
- 2/3 cup Vital Wheat Gluten Flour

Directions

It is not necessary to use vanilla flavored whey protein powder, unflavored is ideal but the vanilla will not contribute much flavor to the mix so if it is what you have on hand, use it.
1. Combine all ingredients and mix thoroughly.
2. Use immediately or store in an airtight container in the refrigerator for up to 1 month. Each recipe makes 9 servings or 3 cups.

3. Each serving size is 1/3 cup.

Nutritional Information
- Protein : 31.3g
- Fat : 4.4g
- Fiber : 3.2g
- Calories : 191

Almond And Coconut Muffin In A Minute

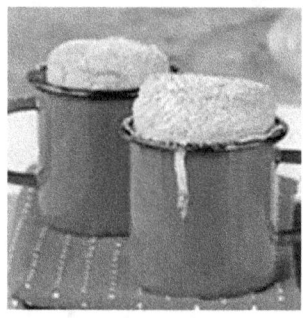

Servings: 1 | **Prep:** 3 m | **Style:** American | **Phase:** 2

Ingredients
- 1/8 cup Almond Meal Flour
- 1/3 tbsp Organic High Fiber Coconut Flour
- 1 tsp Sucralose Based Sweetener (Sugar Substitute)
- 1/2 tsp Cinnamon
- 1/4 tsp Baking Powder (Straight Phosphate, Double Acting)
- 1/8 tsp Salt
- 1 large Egg (Whole)
- 1/3 tbsp Extra Virgin Olive Oil

Directions

1. Place all dry ingredients in a coffee mug. Stir to combine.
2. Add the egg and oil. Stir until thoroughly combined.
3. Microwave for 1 minute. Use a knife if necessary to help remove the muffin from the cup, slice, butter, eat.

Note
- Your MIM can be toasted once it's cooked and topped with cream cheese if you like. Replace the cinnamon with other spices, sugar-free syrup or 1/2 tsp unsweetened cocoa (net carb count will be .2g higher). Add a tablespoon of sour cream for a moister MIM. Change the shape by making it in a bowl.

Nutritional Information
- Protein : 9.7g
- Fat : 16.8g
- Fiber : 3g
- Calories : 207

Almond Muffin In A Minute

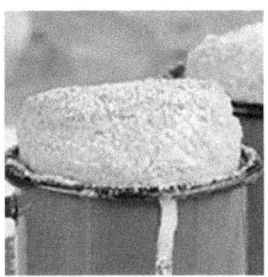

Servings: 1 | Prep: 3 m | Style: American **| Cook time: 1 m**

Ingredients

- 1/4 cup Almond Meal Flour
- 1 tsp Sucralose Based Sweetener (Sugar Substitute)
- 1/4 tsp Baking Powder (Straight Phosphate, Double Acting)
- 1/8 tsp Salt
- 1/2 tsp Cinnamon
- 1 large Egg (Whole)
- 1 tsp Canola Vegetable Oil

Directions
1. Place all dry ingredients in a coffee mug. Stir to combine.
2. Add the egg and oil. Stir until thoroughly combined.
3. Microwave for 1 minute. Use a knife if necessary to help remove the muffin from the cup, slice, butter, eat.

Note
- Your MIM can be toasted once it's cooked and topped with cream cheese if you like. Replace the cinnamon with other spices, sugar-free syrup or 1/2 tsp unsweetened cocoa (net carb count will be .2g higher). Add a tablespoon of sour cream for a moister MIM. Change the shape by making it in a bowl.

Nutritional Information
- Protein : 12.3g
- Fat : 23.4g
- Fiber : 3.7g
- Calories : 279

Almond Protein Pancakes With Blueberries

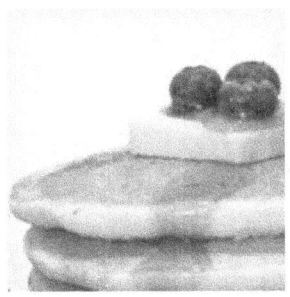

Servings: 1 | **Prep:** 5 m | **Style:** American | **Cook:** 10 m

Ingredients
- 1/16 cup Blanched Almond Flour
- 3/4 large Egg (Whole)
- 1/8 cup dry Whole Grain Soy Flour
- 1/4 tsp Baking Powder (Straight Phosphate, Double Acting)
- 1/2 oz Large or Small Curd Creamed Cottage Cheese
- 2 tbsps Vanilla Whey Protein
- 1/4 cup Fresh Blueberries

Directions
1. Combine the almond flour, protein powder, soy flour and baking powder together. Stir in the beaten egg and cottage cheese until blended.
2. Heat a large nonstick skillet or griddle over medium heat. Lightly grease with butter or canola oil.
3. Using about 1/4 cup per pancake, drop batter onto the skillet. When bubbles begin to form in the middle of each pancake, turn over and cook another 2 minutes or until firm.
4. Serve with blueberries Or add blueberries to the pancake batter before cooking.

Nutritional Information
- Protein : 20.3g
- Fat : 10g
- Fiber : 2.5g
- Calories : 212

Almond Protein Pancakes

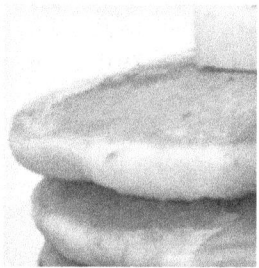

Servings: 4 | **Prep:** 5 m | **Style:** American | **Cook**: 10 m

Ingredients
- 2 oz Vanilla Whey Protein
- 1/4 cup Almond Meal Flour
- 3 tbsps Whole Grain Soy Flour
- 1 tsp Baking Powder (Straight Phosphate, Double Acting)
- 3 large Eggs (Whole)
- 1/3 cup Large or Small Curd Creamed Cottage Cheese

Directions

Serve with almond butter or sugar-free pancake syrup. Garnish with toasted almonds, if desired.

1. Mix the protein powder (1oz is about 4 Tbsp), almond meal, soy flour and baking powder together. Whisk the eggs, then blend together with the cottage cheese (substitute cream cheese if cottage cheese is not on your accepted foods list).
2. Heat a large nonstick skillet or griddle over medium heat. Lightly grease with butter or canola oil.
3. Using about 1/4 cup per pancake, drop batter onto the skillet. When bubbles begin to form in the middle of each pancake, turn over and cook another 2 minutes or until firm.
4. Repeat, keeping pancakes warm in the oven.

Nutritional Information
- Protein : 20g
- Fat : 9.9g
- Fiber : 1.6g
- Calories : 191

Almond-Pineapple Smoothie

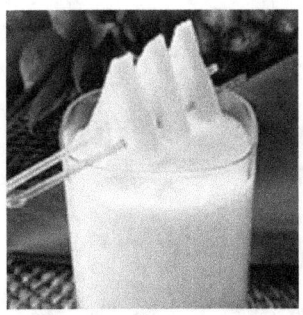

Servings: 1 | **Prep**: 5 m | **Style:** American

Ingredients
- 1/2 cup (8 fl oz) Plain Yogurt (Whole Milk)

- 2 1/2 oz Pineapple
- 20 whole Blanched & Slivered Almonds
- 1/2 cup Pure Almond Milk - Unsweetened Original

Directions
1. Feel free to substitute other fruits or nuts for the pineapple and/or almonds (about 20 whole almonds, 3 Tbsp slivered). Be sure to use fresh pineapple in this smoothie. Canned pineapple is swimming in sugar.
2. Combine the yogurt, pineapple, almonds and almond milk in a blender and purée until smooth and creamy.

Nutritional Information
- Protein : 10.8g
- Fat : 18.6g
- Fiber : 4.2g
- Calories : 280

Almond-Pumpkin Pancakes

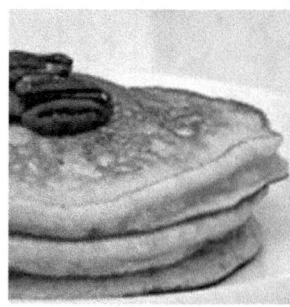

Servings: 6 | **Prep:** 5 m | **Style**: American | **Cook: 10** m

Ingredients

- 4 oz Vanilla Whey Protein
- 4 large Eggs (Whole)
- 1/4 cup Blanched Almond Flour
- 1/4 cup dry Whole Grain Soy Flour
- 1 tsp Baking Powder (Sodium Aluminum Sulfate, Double Acting)
- 1/2 tsp Pumpkin Pie Spice
- 1/4 cup Large or Small Curd Creamed Cottage Cheese
- 1/2 cup Pumpkin (Without Salt, Canned)

Directions

Be sure to use canned pumpkin purée, not pumpkin pie mix (which has added sugar), to make these pancakes. Serve with sugar-free pancake syrup or almond butter.

1. Mix the protein powder, almond meal, soy flour, baking powder and pumpkin pie spice mix in a medium mixing bowl. Stir in the beaten eggs, cottage cheese and pumpkin purée until blended.
2. Heat a large nonstick skillet or griddle over medium heat. Lightly grease skillet with butter or canola oil.
3. Using about 1/4 cup per pancake, drop batter onto the skillet. When bubbles begin to form in the middle of the pancakes, turn and cook another 2 minutes or until firm.
4. Repeat, keeping pancakes warm in the oven before serving.

Nutritional Information
- Protein : 21g
- Fat : 8.4g
- Fiber : 1.8g
- Calories : 183

Almond-Raspberry Smoothie

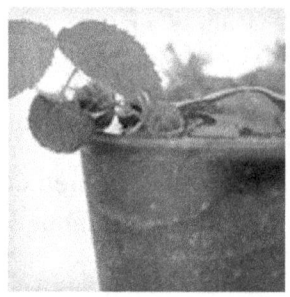

Servings: 1 | **Prep:** 5 m | **Style:** American

Ingredients
- 4 oz Greek Yogurt - Plain (Container)
- 1/2 cup Red Raspberries
- 20 whole Blanched & Slivered Almonds
- 1/2 cup Pure Almond Milk - Unsweetened Original

Directions
1. Feel free to come up with your own combination of other berries and nuts for this protein-packed smoothie. If you use frozen raspberries, make sure they contain no added sugar.
2. Combine the yogurt, raspberries, almonds and almond milk in a blender and purée until smooth and creamy.

Nutritional Information
- Protein : 18.1g
- Fat : 17.8g
- Fiber : 7.1g
- Calories : 291

Ancho Macho Chili

Servings: 10 | **Prep:** 10 m | **Style:** American | **Cook:** 165 m

Ingredients
- 5 lbs Beef Top Sirloin (Trimmed to 1/8" Fat)
- 2 tsps Salt
- 1/2 tsp Black Pepper
- 3 tbsps Extra Virgin Olive Oil
- 1 medium (2-1/2" dia) Onions
- 2 tsps Garlic
- 3 tbsps Chili Powder
- 14 1/2 oz Red Tomatoes (with Green Chilies, Canned)
- 6 fl ozs Red Table Wine

Directions

Cooking evaporates alcohol, which is why this recipe is suitable for Induction despite the red wine. But feel free to use chicken broth instead. Jarred roasted garlic cloves can be found in the produce section of most supermarkets or simply mince a whole clove of garlic.

1. Heat oven to 325°F.
2. Season beef with salt and pepper. Heat 1 1/2 teaspoons oil in a Dutch oven over high heat. Add one-third of the beef and brown on all sides, about 1 minutes per side.
3. Transfer to a bowl and repeat two more times with beef and oil.

4. Chop the onion and add to a Dutch oven preheated with the remaining 1 1/2 teaspoons oil. Cook onion and garlic until lightly browned. Stir in chile powder, tomatoes and wine; bring to a simmer. Return beef and accumulated juices to Dutch oven. Cover and bake 2 1/2 hours, stirring once halfway through cooking time, until beef is very tender. One serving is about 3/4-1 cup.

Nutritional Information
- Protein : 43.9g
- Fat : 12.4g
- Fiber : 1.4g
- Calories :325

Apple Muffins With Cinnamon-Pecan Streusel

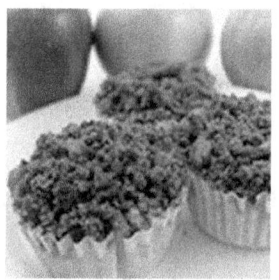

Servings: 8 | **Prep:** 15 m | **Style:** American | **Cook:** 25 m

Ingredients
- 1 2/3 cups Almond Meal Flour
- 1/2 cup half Pecans
- 6 1/2 tsps Cinnamon
- 1/3 tsp Salt

- 24 tsps Erythritol
- 1 pinch Stevia
- 2 tbsps Unsalted Butter Stick
- 2 large Eggs (Whole)
- 1/4 cup Coconut Milk Unsweetened
- 2 tsps Vanilla Extract
- 2 tbsps Organic High Fiber Coconut Flour
- 1 tsp Baking Powder (Straight Phosphate, Double Acting)
- 2/3 cup quartered or chopped Apple

Directions
1. Preheat oven to 350 F. Prepare a muffin tin with 8 cupcake papers.
2. Combine 2/3 cup almond flour, chopped pecans, 2 tablespoons cinnamon, 1/8 teaspoon salt, 2 tablespoons granular sugar substitute (eryhtritol), a pinch of stevia and 2 tablespoons melted butter in a small bowl. Mix with a fork until it begins to crumble. Set aside while making the muffin batter.
3. For the muffins: whisk together the eggs, 1/4 cup coconut milk, 2 teaspoons vanilla, 6 tablespoons granular sugar substitute (erythritol), a pinch of stevia, and 1/2 teaspoon ground cinnamon. Add 1 cup almond flour, 2 tablespoons coconut flour, 1/4 teaspoon salt and 1 teaspoon baking powder; mix to combine then fold in 2/3 cup finely chopped apples.
4. Divide into muffin 8 wells topping each with about 2 tablespoons of the struesal. Bake for 25 minutes, remove from oven and allow to sit for 10-20 minutes to cool before removing. These may be eaten immediately or stored in an airtight container in the refrigerator for up to 1 week.

Nutritional Information
- Protein : 7.5g

- Fat : 20.6g
- Fiber : 5.1g
- Calories : 242

Asian Beef Salad Single Serving

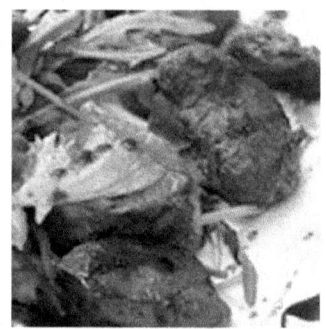

Servings: 1 | **Prep:** 720 m | **Style:** American | **Cook:** 5 m

Ingredients
- 1/2 clove Garlic
- 1/2 tbsp Tamari Soybean Sauce
- 1/4 tbsp Sodium and Sugar Free Rice Vinegar
- 1/4 tsp Sesame Oil
- 1/8 tsp Sucralose Based Sweetener (Sugar Substitute)
- 1/8 tsp Curry Powder
- 1/16 tsp Ginger
- 4 1/4 oz Beef Top Sirloin (Trimmed to 1/8" Fat, Choice Grade)
- 3/4 cup Spring Mix Salad
- 1/2 tbsp Canola Vegetable Oil

- 1/4 large (2-1/4 per lb, approx 3-3/4" long, 3" dia) Sweet Red Peppers
- 2 oz Waterchestnuts
- 1 large Scallions or Spring Onion

Directions

Note: Because only half of the marinade is used in this recipe for the salad dressing and the rest is used as a marinade and discarded, please double the first six ingredients. (The nutritionals shown are correct.) For added flavor, use dark (toasted) sesame oil instead of regular sesame oil.

1. Mix green onions, garlic, soy sauce, rice wine vinegar, sesame oil and sugar substitute in a small bowl. Pour half into a resealable plastic bag; add steak and marinate overnight in the refrigerator.
2. To remaining soy sauce mixture, add curry powder and ginger. Heat canola oil in a large skillet over high heat until very hot.
3. Drain beef and discard marinade; quickly stir-fry beef 2 to 3 minutes in hot oil for medium doneness. Transfer to a large mixing bowl. Add salad greens, bell pepper, water chestnuts and reserved soy dressing. Toss to coat and serve immediately.

Nutritional Information
- Protein : 29.5g
- Fat : 13.3g
- Fiber : 4.1g
- Calories :295

Atkins Cinnamon Pie Crust

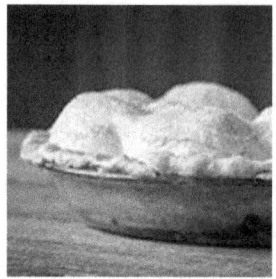

Servings: 8 | **Prep:** 10 m | **Style:** American

Ingredients
- 1/4 tsp Salt
- 1 tsp Sucralose Based Sweetener (Sugar Substitute)
- 1 tsp Cinnamon
- 1/2 cup Unsalted Butter Stick
- 3 3/4 servings All Purpose Low-Carb Baking Mix
- 2 tbsps Tap Water

Directions
1. Use the Atkins recipe to make All Purpose Low-Carb Baking Mix. You will need 1 1/4 cups to make one pie crust.
2. Pulse the baking mix, salt, sugar substitute, and cinnamon in a food processor to incorporate; add butter and pulse until mixture resembles a coarse meal, about 30 seconds. Pulse in water until dough just comes together, about 30 seconds (add up to 1 more tablespoon if necessary).
3. Transfer dough to a sheet of plastic wrap; form into a a disk about 6 inches in diameter. Wrap tightly in plastic; refrigerate until firm, about 30 minutes.

4. Roll and bake as directed in pie recipe. Makes 1 pie crust.

Nutritional Information
- Protein : 14.8g
- Fat : 13.6g
- Fiber : 1.7g
- Calories : 193

Atkins Cuisine Biscuits

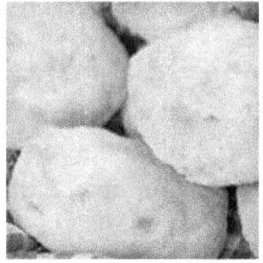

Servings: 18 | **Prep:** 25 m | **Style:** American | **Cook:** 20 m

Ingredients
- 1 1/2 tsps Baking Powder (Straight Phosphate, Double Acting)
- 3/4 tsp Salt
- 1 individual packet Sucralose Based Sweetener (Sugar Substitute)
- 1/2 cup Unsalted Butter Stick
- 6 servings All Purpose Low-Carb Baking Mix
- 1 cup Heavy Cream

Directions
1. Preheat oven to 425°F degrees.
2. Blend together 2 cups low-carb baking mix, baking powder, sugar substitute and salt in a large mixing bowl.
3. Cut butter into small chunks and add to the dry ingredients, using a pastry blender or your fingertips to work until the mixture resembles coarse crumbs. Do not over-mix.
4. Pour in heavy cream and stir lightly.
5. Coat cutting board with olive oil spray. Using a spatula, transfer the dough to a cutting board. Coat hands with oil spray and lightly knead dough a few times until blended. Do not over knead.
6. Pat out dough into a circle 1/2 3/4-inch thick. Using a biscuit cutter with a 2¼-inch diameter, form biscuits. Make an extra biscuit out of scraps instead of re-rolling the dough.
7. Place biscuits on a baking sheet coated with oil spray. Brush tops with melted butter, if desired.
8. Bake 15 -18 minutes or until golden brown.
9. Remove biscuits from oven and place on a wire rack to cool.

Nutritional Information
- Protein : 10.7g
- Fat : 11.5g
- Fiber : 1.1g
- Calories : 155

Atkins Cuisine Pancakes

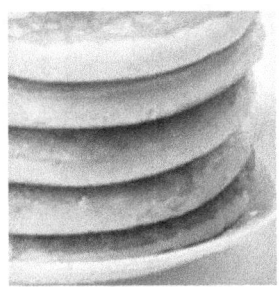

Servings: 10 | **Prep:** 5 m | **Style:** American | **Cook:** 15 m

Ingredients
- 1 individual packet Sucralose Based Sweetener (Sugar Substitute)
- 1 large Egg (Whole)
- 2 tsps Baking Powder (Straight Phosphate, Double Acting)
- 1/4 tsp Salt
- 1 cup Cream (Half & Half)
- 3 servings All Purpose Low-Carb Baking Mix

Directions
1. Blend together 1 cup baking mix, sugar substitute, baking powder and salt in a large mixing bowl.
2. Add the half and half and egg. Whisk batter. Let the mixture sit for at least 5 minutes to activate the baking powder.
3. Coat the griddle with olive oil spray. Over medium heat, cook 4 pancakes at a time. When bubbles appear on the top and the edges are firm, flip the pancakes and cook another 2 3 minutes. Keep warm in the oven.
4. Repeat with remaining pancakes.

Nutritional Information
- Protein : 7.4g
- Fat : 4.6g
- Fiber : 1.8g
- Calories : 85

Atkins Cuisine Pie Crust

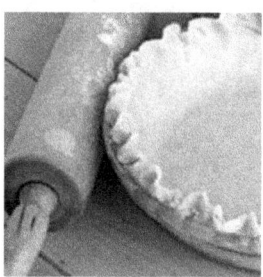

Servings: 8 | **Prep:** 10 m | **Style:** American

Ingredients
- 1/3 cup 100% Stone Ground Whole Wheat Pastry Flour
- 1/3 cup Whole Grain Soy Flour
- 2 oz Vital Wheat Gluten
- 3 tbsps Plain Wheat Germ
- 1/2 tsp Salt
- 1/2 cup Unsalted Butter Stick
- 1 tbsp Tap Water

Directions
1. In a food processor, pulse flours, wheat gluten, germ, salt and butter until mixture resembles a coarse meal. Slowly add water and continue pulsing until the dough begins to come

together. Turn onto a sheet of plastic wrap, form into a ball and cover with plastic. Flatten to a 7-inch disc and chill in the freezer for 15 minutes.
2. Roll dough out between 2 sheets of plastic wrap to a 12-inch circle (if needed, sprinkle on 1/2 teaspoon wheat gluten flour per side to facilitate rolling). Remove the top sheet of plastic and invert onto a 9-inch pie plate. Center dough and press onto the bottom and sides of plate. Remove plastic, roll under the edges and crimp decoratively. Chill in the freezer for 15 minutes.
3. Use unbaked crust as indicated in recipe of your choice. Or for a prebaked crust, preheat oven to 400° F. Prick the bottom and corners of the pie shell with a fork. Line the pie shell with foil, fill halfway with pie weights or dried beans and turn the foil over to cover the pastry edge. Bake for 16 minutes. Remove the foil and weights, cover loosely with foil and bake an additional 4 to 6 minutes or until golden. Cool on a rack for 20 minutes before using.
4. Makes 8 servings.

Nutritional Information
- Protein : 7.9g
- Fat : 12.7g
- Fiber : 1.6g
- Calories : 173

Atkins Cuisine Waffles

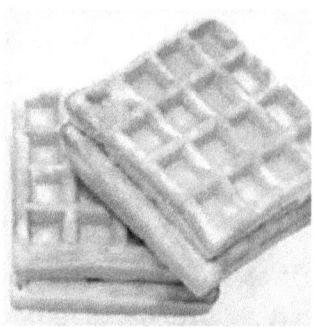

Servings: 5 | **Prep:** 10 m | **Style:** American | **Cook:** 10 m

Ingredients
- 1 individual packet Sucralose Based Sweetener (Sugar Substitute)
- 1 large Egg (Whole)
- 2 tsps Baking Powder (Straight Phosphate, Double Acting)
- 1/4 tsp Salt
- 1 cup Cream (Half & Half)
- 3 servings All Purpose Low-Carb Baking Mix

Directions

Use the Atkins recipe to make All Purpose Low-Carb Baking Mix for this recipe. This recipe makes 5 waffles. Assuming your waffle iron makes 4 servings, use four-fifths of the batter and then make a single waffle with the remaining batter. Freeze extra waffles and just pop in the toaster before serving.

1. In a large bowl, blend together 1 cup baking mix, baking powder, sugar substitute and salt.
2. In another large bowl, mix the half-and-half and beaten egg.
3. Add dry ingredients to the liquid ingredients and whisk batter until any lumps are removed. Don't overbeat.
4. Let the mixture sit for at least 5 minutes to activate the baking powder.
5. Heat the waffle iron and pour the batter in the center of the waffle iron.
6. Close the top and cook waffles for about 1 1 1/2 minutes or until golden brown.
7. Repeat with last waffle.

Nutritional Information
- Protein : 21.4g
- Fat : 9g
- Fiber : 1.9g
- Calories : 193

Bacon, Avocado And Jack Cheese Omelets With Fresh Salsa

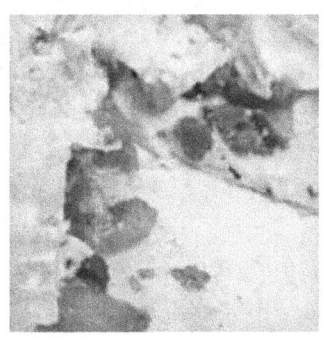

Servings: 2 | **Prep:** 10 m | **Style:** American | **Cook:** 10 m

Ingredients
- 1 medium whole (2-3/5" dia) Red Tomato
- 3 medium (4-1/8" long) Scallions or Spring Onions
- 1/2 Jalapeno Peppers
- 1 oz Cilantro
- 1 tbsp Fresh Lime Juice
- 4 large Eggs (Whole)
- 1 fl oz Tap Water
- 3 medium slice (yield after cooking) Bacon
- 1 tbsp Unsalted Butter Stick
- 1/2 California Avocados
- 1 cup shredded Monterey Jack Cheese

Directions
1. Prepare salsa: Chop the tomatoes; finely chop the green onions and jalapeno (de-seed if you would like less heat). In small bowl, combine tomato, green onions, jalapeño, cilantro and lime juice and mix well. Season to taste with salt and pepper. Set aside.
2. In medium bowl, whisk eggs with water and season with salt and pepper. Prepare bacon, cook thoroughly, crumble and set aside.
3. Melt half the butter in a small nonstick skillet over medium-high heat. When foam subsides, add half the egg mixture. Tilt pan to coat bottom and cook 1 minute, until almost set. Sprinkle half the omelet with half the crumbled bacon, avocado and cheese and cook 1 minute.
4. Fold empty half of omelet over filling and slide omelet onto a plate. Keep warm.
5. Repeat with remaining butter, egg mixture, bacon, avocado and cheese. Serve with salsa.

Nutritional Information
- Protein : 33g
- Fat : 42.5g
- Fiber : 3.9g
- Calories : 553

Baked Eggs And Asparagus

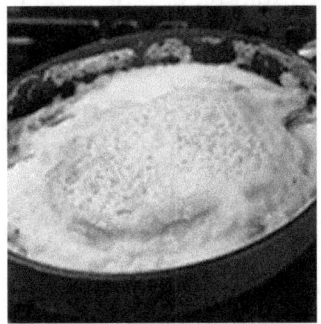

Servings: 1 | **Prep:** 5 m | **Style:** American | **Cook:** 10 m

Ingredients
- 8 spear small (5" long or less) Asparagus
- 1/4 cup Heavy Cream
- 2 large Eggs (Whole)
- 2 tbsps Almond Meal Flour
- 1 tbsp Parmesan Cheese (Shredded)
- 1/8 tsp Garlic
- 1/8 tsp Black Pepper

Directions

1. Preheat oven to 400°F. Prepare a small oven safe casserole or 4-inch by 3-inch dish with a little bit of oil. Set aside.
2. Boil the asparagus spears for 2 minutes until tender-crisp. Drain and run under cold water then pat dry. Arrange in the prepared baking dish.
3. Pour cream over the asparagus and then crack two eggs on top.
4. In a small bowl blend together the almond meal, Parmesan cheese, garlic and black pepper. Sprinkle over the eggs and place in the oven. Cook for 5-10 minutes depending upon how you like your eggs cooked. Longer time will result in a firmer yolk. The cream will puff over the edges of the eggs and the topping should be golden brown and fragrant.

Nutritional Information
- Protein : 20.8g
- Fat : 40.4g
- Fiber : 4g
- Calories : 471

Basque Eggs With Ham, Tomatoes And Bell Peppers

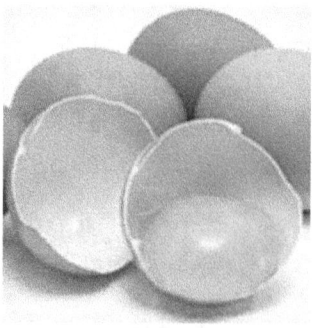

Servings: 6 | **Prep:** 30 m | **Style:** American | **Cook:** 12 mins

Ingredients
- 3 tbsps Extra Virgin Olive Oil
- 1 medium (2-1/2" dia) Onions
- 8 oz Roasted Bell Peppers
- 2 plums Red Tomatoes
- 5 1/2 tbsps Basil
- 1/4 tsp Red or Cayenne Pepper
- 12 large Eggs (Whole)
- 6 tbsps Unsalted Butter Stick
- 6 oz boneless, cooked Fresh Ham
- 3 tsps Garlic

Directions
1. Heat oil in large heavy skillet over medium heat. Sauté onion 5 minutes, until softened; add garlic and cook 1 minute more.
2. Add roasted peppers, tomatoes, and cayenne. Cover and cook 10 minutes, until vegetables are very soft, stirring occasionally.
3. Uncover and simmer over medium heat until sauce is thick, about 10 minutes, stirring often. Season to taste with salt and pepper. (Mixture can be made up to 2 days ahead and reheated).
4. In large bowl, beat eggs until blended. In large nonstick skillet, melt butter over low heat. Add eggs and basil. Cook, stirring constantly with rubber spatula, 12 minutes, until soft curds form and eggs are barely set.
5. Add pepper mixture and ham; stir just until mixed.

Nutritional Information
- Protein : 19.6g
- Fat : 30.2g
- Fiber : 1.1g
- Calories : 379

Béchamel Sauce

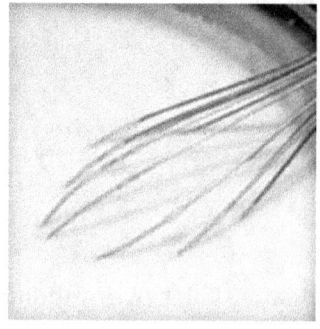

Servings: 6 | **Prep**: 10 m | **Style:** American | **Cook**: 20 m

Ingredients
- 1 cup Heavy Cream
- 1 cup Tap Water
- 2 tbsps chopped Onions
- 1 tsp Salt
- 1/8 tsp Black Pepper
- 1/8 tsp Nutmeg (Ground)
- 3 tsps Thick-It-Up
- 1 tbsp Unsalted Butter Stick

Directions

Béchamel is a mild sauce that can be used in soufflés or simmered with finely chopped vegetables or meats. Traditionally thickened with a mixture of flour and fat, our version uses heavy cream and a low-carb thickener instead. Each serving is 1/4 cup.

1. Combine cream, water, white onion, salt, pepper and nutmeg in a small saucepan over medium heat; bring to a simmer. Remove from heat; let stand for 15 minutes.
2. Strain cream mixture; return to saucepan over medium heat. Whisk in 1 tablespoon Thick-It-Up thickener; cook until sauce thickens, about 3 minutes.
3. Remove from heat; swirl in butter until melted. Use immediately

Nutritional Information
- Protein : 0.9g
- Fat : 16.7g
- Fiber : 1.1g
- Calories : 163

Beef Huevos Rancheros On Canadian Bacon

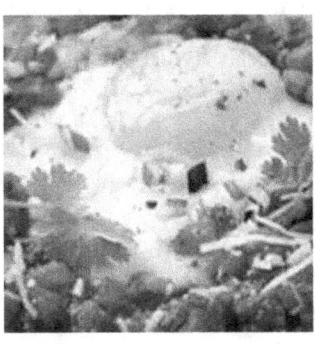

Servings: 4 | **Prep**: 10 m | **Style**: American | **Cook**: 20 m

Ingredients
- 6 oz Ground Beef (80% Lean / 20% Fat)
- 1/2 cup Green Chili Peppers (Canned)
- 1/4 tsp Garlic Powder
- 1 tsp Chili Powder
- 1/4 tsp Cumin
- 1/4 tsp leaf Oregano
- 1/4 tsp Salt
- 1/4 tsp Black Pepper
- 4 slices Canadian Bacon
- 4 large Eggs (Whole)
- 1/2 cup shredded Cheddar Cheese
- 4 sprigs Cilantro

Directions

The directions for this dish call for scrambled eggs, but you can also serve them fried or poached.

1. In a greased medium skillet, brown the beef over medium heat.
2. Stir in chiles, garlic powder, chili powder, cumin, oregano, salt and pepper. Cook 5-10 minutes to blend the flavors.
3. Lay the Canadian bacon slices over the top of the beef mixture to warm. Remove pan from heat and set aside.
4. In another skillet, scramble eggs until firm.
5. Place 1 piece of Canadian bacon on each plate, top with a quarter of the beef mixture and a quarter of the eggs. Sprinkle with cheese and chopped cilantro.

Nutritional Information

- Protein : 23.1g
- Fat : 15g
- Fiber : 0.6g
- Calories : 244

Beef Sautéed With Green Bell Pepper And Onions Topped With Cheese

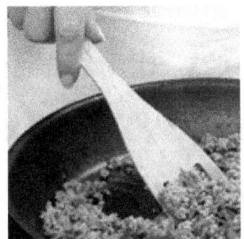

Servings: 1 | **Prep:** 5 m | **Style:** American | **Cook:** 10 m

Ingredients
- 1/4 cup chopped Onions
- 1 tbsp Extra Virgin Olive Oil
- 1/2 cup chopped Green Sweet Pepper
- 1/2 cup shredded Cheddar Cheese
- 5 oz Ground Beef (80% Lean / 20% Fat)

Directions
1. Sauté ground beef in a skillet over medium-high heat with small amount of cooking oil for 1-2 minutes. Add green bell pepper and white onions.
2. Sauté until beef is browned and the peppers and onions are soft. Add salt and pepper to taste.
3. Drain off any excess fat and put onto a serving plate. Sprinkle cheese on top and allow to melt. Serve immediately.

Nutritional Information
- Protein : 43.5g
- Fat : 47.1g
- Fiber : 2g
- Calories : 628

Bell Pepper Rings Filled With Egg And Mozzarella With Fruit

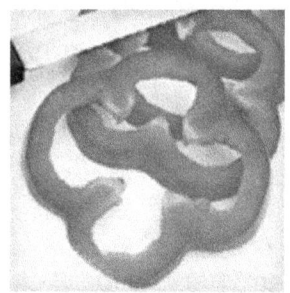

Servings: 1 | **Prep:** 10 m | **Style:** American | **Cook:** 5 m

Ingredients
- 1/4 cup shredded Whole Milk Mozzarella Cheese
- 1 tsp Extra Virgin Olive Oil
- 1/4 small (6" to 6-7/8" long) Bananas
- 1/4 small (2-1/2" dia) (approx 4 per lb) Apples
- 1/2 fruit Kiwi Fruit
- 2 large Eggs (Whole)
- 1/4 cup Raspberries

- 1/2 medium (approx 2-3/4" long, 2-1/2" dia) Sweet Red Peppers

Directions
1. Cut bell pepper into two 1- inch rounds.
2. Place rounds in a skillet with a small amount of oil over medium high heat.
3. Crack 1 egg into each round, cook for 2 minutes then add 1-2 Tbsp water to pan and steam the egg and pepper for 3-5 additional minutes until the egg is cooked to your liking.
4. Top with cheese. Leave in the pan and cover for about 1 minute to melt cheese.
5. Combine the fruits and serve with the pepper rings.

Nutritional Information
- Protein : 19.9g
- Fat : 20.6g
- Fiber : 5.8g
- Calories : 361

Blackberry Smoothie

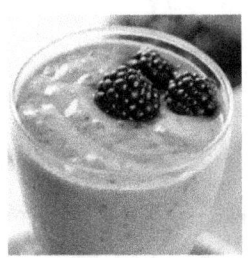

Servings: 1 | **Prep:** 5 m | **Style:** American

Ingredients
- 1/4 cup Frozen Blackberries
- 1 cup Coconut Milk Unsweetened
- 1/4 tsp Cinnamon
- 1/2 tsp Vanilla Extract
- 1 scoop Vanilla Whey Protein
- 1/16 tsp Allspice Ground
- 1/16 cup Organic 100% Whole Ground Golden Flaxseed Meal

Directions
1. For this recipe unsweetened coconut, almond or soy milk may be used. Combine the frozen balckberries, milk of choice, protein powder, vanilla and spices in a blender. Blend until smooth.

Nutritional Information
- Protein : 21.8g
- Fat : 9.8g
- Fiber : 5.8g
- Calories : 221

Blueberry Cloud Muffin

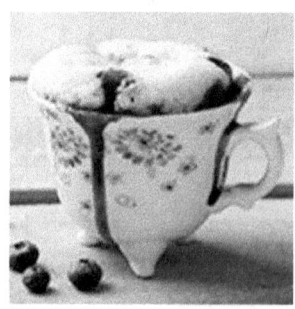

Servings: 1 | **Prep:** 1 m | **Style**: American | **Cook:** 1 m

Ingredients
- 1 oz Cream Cheese
- 1 large Egg
- 2 tbsps Vanilla Whey Protein
- 1/4 tsp Baking Powder (Sodium Aluminum Sulfate, Double Acting)
- 1/8 tsp Nutmeg (Ground)
- 1/4 cup Blueberries

Directions
1. Place cream cheese in a microwave safe mug. Heat for 10-15 seconds (enough to warm the cream cheese but not to fully melt it).
2. Add the egg and whisk it with the cream cheese.
3. Add the whey protein powder (use a protein powder that has 1g NC or less per serving, one serving is about 1 oz), baking powder, and nutmeg; whisk to combine. Add the blueberries mixing to combine. Heat the mug in the microwave for 1 min and 20 seconds (the blueberries need additional time to cook since they contain so much moisture. Microwave times vary so you may need to increase the time by 10-20 seconds if it does not cook through. Remove muffin by turning over onto a plate. Run a knife around the inside of the mug to more easily release it.

Nutritional Information
- Protein : 19.2g
- Fat : 15.1g
- Fiber : 0.9g
- Calories : 242

Breakfast Burrito

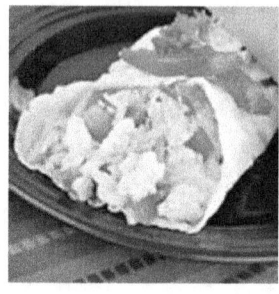

Servings: 2 | **Prep**: 15 m | **Style:** American | **Cook:** 5 m

Ingredients
- 1/2 tsp Salt
- 1/4 tsp Red or Cayenne Pepper
- 1 tbsp Canola Vegetable Oil
- 4 large Eggs (Whole)
- 3 tbsps Sweet Red Peppers
- 2 tbsps chopped Scallions or Spring Onions
- 1 Jalapeno Pepper
- 2 tortillas Low Carb Tortillas
- 1/8 tsp Tabasco Sauce
- 2 oz Salsa

Directions
1. Whisk eggs, salt and cayenne together in a bowl.
2. In a medium skillet over medium heat, toast tortillas 1 minute per side until brown in spots; set aside and cover with foil to keep warm.

3. In the same skillet add oil, red pepper, scallion whites and jalapeno. Cook until vegetables are softened, about 3 minutes.
4. Add eggs and continue to cook, stirring, until eggs are set, about 2 minutes.
5. Place tortillas on plates. Divide eggs between tortillas, season with hot sauce and gently roll up.
6. Serve with salsa and scallion greens.

Note: This can be made with a whole wheat or low-carb tortilla if you are in an acceptable phase. The whole wheat tortillas used here have 20g NC each so be sure to adjust the NC to the tortilla you are using. Low-carb tortillas typically have less NC than the whole wheat.

Nutritional Information
- Protein : 17.8g
- Fat : 19.2g
- Fiber : 5g
- Calories : 281

Breakfast Mexi Peppers

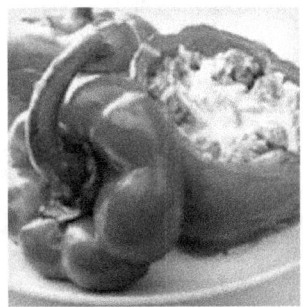

Servings: 4 | **Prep:** 30 m | **Style:** American | **Cook:** 30 m

Ingredients
- 4 oz Pork and Beef Chorizo
- 4 oz Ground Beef (80% Lean / 20% Fat)
- 1/2 cup chopped Onions
- 1/4 cup shredded Cheddar Cheese
- 3 large Eggs (Whole)
- 2 medium (approx 2-3/4" long, 2-1/2" dia) Sweet Red Peppers

Directions
1. Preheat oven to 400°F. Line a baking sheet with foil.
2. Cook chorizo, stirring to break up lumps, until browned. Drain excess fat.
3. Place chorizo and ground beef in mixing bowl and combine with the onion, cheese and eggs.
4. Cut peppers in half lengthwise. Scoop out seeds and cut away ribs.
5. Fill each pepper with one-quarter of the meat mixture. Place on the prepared baking sheet. Bake for 25 30 minutes and serve hot.

Nutritional Information
- Protein : 21.3g
- Fat : 20.1g
- Fiber : 1.5g
- Calories : 298

Breakfast Sausage Sautéed With Red And Green Bell Peppers

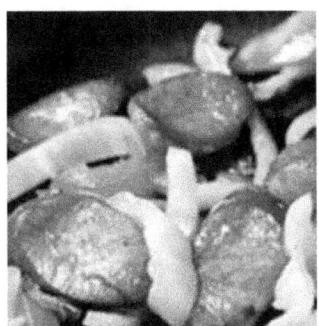

Servings: 1 | **Prep:** 5 m | **Style:** Other | **Cook:** 10 m

Ingredients
- 1 tsp Canola Vegetable Oil
- 4 link cookeds Turkey Breakfast Sausage
- 1/4 large (2.25 per pound, approx 3-3/4" long, 3" dia) Red Sweet Pepper
- 1/4 large (2.25 per pound, approx 3-3/4" long, 3" dia) Green Sweet Pepper
- 1 slice (1 oz) Monterey Jack Cheese

Directions
1. Heat a skillet with 1 teaspoon oil over medium-high heat.
2. Crumble the sausage link or leave whole and slice after cooking. Sauté until just beginning to brown. About 3 minutes. Add in red and green bell peppers. Cook until sausage is browned and peppers are softened, about 5 minutes.
3. Sprinkle cheese on top and allow to melt 1-2 minutes. Serve immediately.

Nutritional Information
- Protein : 25.7g
- Fat : 33.4g
- Fiber : 1.5g
- Calories : 408

Buttermilk Cinnamon Waffles

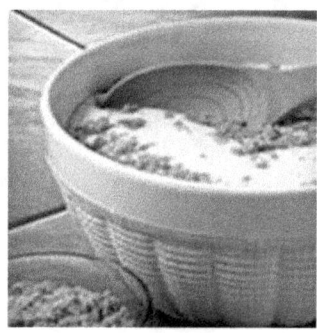

Servings: 8 | **Prep:** 10 m | **Style:** American | **Cook:** 4 m

Ingredients
- 1 cup Whole Grain Soy Flour
- 2 tbsps Sucralose Based Sweetener (Sugar Substitute)
- 2 tsps Cinnamon
- 3 tsps Baking Powder (Straight Phosphate, Double Acting)
- 1/2 tsp Baking Soda
- 3/4 cup Buttermilk (Reduced Fat, Cultured)
- 6 tbsps Unsalted Butter Stick
- 3 large Eggs (Whole)
- 1 1/2 oz Sugar Free French Vanilla Syrup
- 1/2 cup Tap Water
- 1/3 second spray Original Canola Cooking Spray

Directions
1. Heat waffle iron per manufacturers instructions.
2. Whisk together soy flour, sugar substitute, cinnamon, baking powder and baking soda. Add buttermilk, butter, eggs and syrup and stir until well blended (batter will be stiff).
3. Add cold water 1 tablespoon (8 tbsp in a 1/2 cup) at a time until batter is easily spoonable and spreadable, about the consistency of a thick pancake batter.
4. Spray waffle iron with oil spray. Place approximately 3 tablespoons of batter in center of a waffle iron.
5. Cook according to manufacturer's instructions until crisp and dark golden brown.
6. Repeat with remaining batter. Serve warm. Enjoy!

Nutritional Information
- Protein : 6.9g
- Fat : 13g
- Fiber : 1.4g
- Calories : 166

California Breakfast Burrito

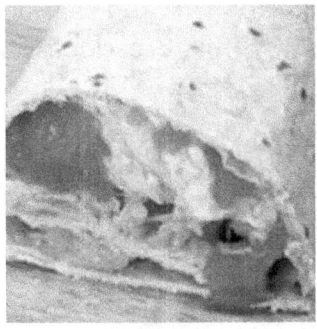

Servings: 4 | **Prep**: 20 m | **Style**: Mexican | **Cook**: 5 m

Ingredients
- 4 tortillas Low Carb Tortillas
- 1 tbsp Canola Vegetable Oil
- 3 large Scallions or Spring Onions
- 4 oz Green Chili Peppers (Canned)
- 1 medium whole (2-3/5" dia) Red Tomato
- 1/2 tsp Salt
- 1/4 tsp Black Pepper
- 8 large Eggs (Whole)
- 1/8 tsp Red or Cayenne Pepper
- 9 sprigs Cilantro (Coriander)
- 1/2 cup shredded Cheddar Cheese
- 1 serving Tomatillo Salsa

Directions

Use 1/4 cup total of the Atkins recipe for Tomatillo Salsa.

1. Heat oven to 325° F.
2. Wrap tortillas in foil and heat in oven 5-10 minutes. Chop tomatoes and dice green onions.
3. In a medium nonstick skillet, heat oil over medium-high heat. Add green onions, chiles, tomato, salt and pepper. Sauté for 3 minutes.
4. Push mixture to side of pan. Add eggs and cayenne to skillet. Cook, 1-2 minutes, stirring occasionally with rubber spatula, until soft, creamy curds form.
5. Stir vegetable mixture into eggs.
6. Divide mixture among warm tortillas, sprinkle with cilantro, one tablespoon of salsa and 2 tablespoons cheese. Roll up tortillas.

Nutritional Information
- Protein : 21.5g

- Fat : 21.1g
- Fiber : 5.5g
- Calories : 317

Canadian Bacon, Cheddar And Tomato Stacks

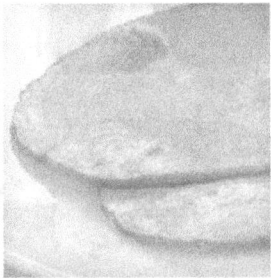

Servings: 1 | **Prep:** 5 m | **Style:** American | **Cook:** 5 m

Ingredients
- 2 slices (6 per 6-oz pkg.) Canadian-Style Bacon (Cured)
- 1 large whole (3" dia) Red Tomato
- 1/4 cup shredded Cheddar Cheese

Directions
1. In a skillet over medium-high heat sauté the Canadian bacon until nicely browned and warmed through.
2. Top with a slice of tomato and then cheddar while still in the pan. Cover with a lid and allow to steam with a teaspoon of water for about 1 minute to heat the tomato and melt the cheese.
3. Plate and serve immediately.

Nutritional Information
- Protein : 20.4g

- Fat : 13.7g
- Fiber : 2.2g
- Calories : 236

Carrot-Zucchini Latkes

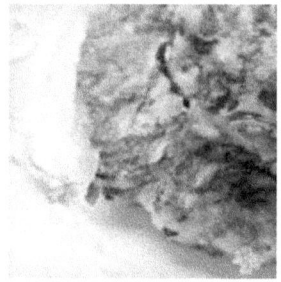

Servings: 8 | **Prep:** 15 m | **Style:** Middle Eastern | **Cook:** 40 m

Ingredients
- 12 oz Zucchini
- 3/4 tsp Salt
- 5 medium Carrots
- 1 small Onion
- 4 large Eggs (Whole)
- 1/2 tsp Black Pepper
- 1/2 cup Canola Vegetable Oil
- 1 1/2 servings Atkins Cuisine Bread

Directions

Use the Atkins recipe to make Atkins Cuisine Bread for this recipe.

1. Heat oven to 300°F. Set a rack on a baking sheet.
2. Grate zucchini in a food processor fitted with shredding blade or with a box grater, using the side with the largest holes. Transfer to a bowl; sprinkle with 1/4 teaspoon of the salt and toss. Let stand while you prepare the remaining ingredients.
3. Grate carrots and white onion in food processor or with the grater. Transfer to a large bowl.
4. Put bread on a baking sheet and toast in the oven until dried out, 10 to 14 minutes. Leave oven on. Transfer bread to food processor and pulverize to make crumbs. Add crumbs, eggs, remaining 1/2 teaspoon salt and pepper to carrots. Transfer zucchini to a clean dish towel and squeeze out excess liquid. Add zucchini to carrot mixture and stir well to combine.
5. Heat 1/2 cup of canola oil (may need to add more during cooking) in a large skillet over medium heat until very hot. Drop batter by heaping tablespoons into oil and flatten to 3-inch pancakes; do not crowd pan. Cook until golden brown, 3 to 4 minutes per side. Transfer to paper towels to drain; then set on prepared baking sheet and keep latkes warm in oven. Repeat, adding more oil if necessary, making a total of 24 latkes. Serve with sour cream or a squeeze of lemon (optional).

Nutritional Information
- Protein : 5g
- Fat : 17.1g
- Fiber : 1.9g
- Calories : 197

Cheddar Omelet With Avocado And Salsa

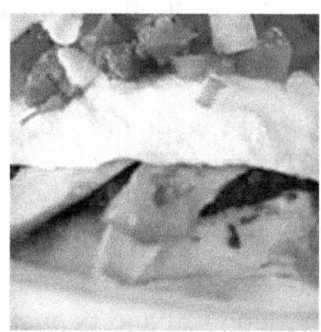

Servings: 1 | **Prep:** 5 m | **Style:** American | **Cook:** 10 m

Ingredients
- 1 tsp Canola Vegetable Oil
- 2 large Eggs (Whole)
- 1 oz Cheddar Cheese
- 1/2 fruit without skin and seed California Avocados
- 1 oz Salsa

Directions
1. Heat oil in a nonstick skillet over medium high heat. Add slightly beaten eggs to skillet. Cook 3 minutes, flip over, cook other side for 2 minutes.
2. Add shredded Cheddar and avocado to half of the omelet. Flip other half over top. Cook an additional 1-2 minutes to melt cheese.
3. Top with salsa and serve immediately.

Nutritional Information
- Protein : 20.8g
- Fat : 33.6g

- Fiber : 5g
- Calories : 419

Cheddar Omelet With Sautéed Onions And Shiitake Mushrooms

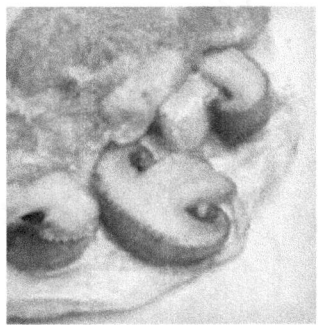

Servings: 1 | **Prep:** 5 m | **Style:** American | **Cook:** 8 m

Ingredients
- 1/4 cup shredded Cheddar Cheese
- 1/3 cup chopped Onions
- 1 tsp Canola Vegetable Oil
- 2 large Eggs (Whole)
- 1/4 cup Shiitake Mushrooms

Directions
- Heat oil in a nonstick skillet or omelet pan over medium-high heat. Add onions and mushrooms. Sauté for about 5 minutes until onions are translucent and mushrooms are soft. Remove from pan and set aside.
- Add eggs to the skillet. Cook 3 minutes, lifting the edges of the egg to allow uncooked eggs to flow over and cook. Flip over and cook another 2 minutes.

- Add onions and mushrooms to half of omelet and top with cheese. Fold other half over and cook 1 -2 minutes more to melt cheese. Serve immediately.

Nutritional Information
- Protein : 21.5g
- Fat : 23.9g
- Fiber : 2.3g
- Calories :339

Cheddar Omelet With Sautéed Onions

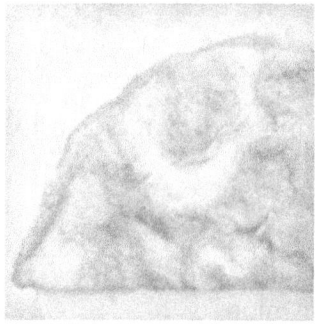

Servings: 1 | **Prep:** 5 m | **Style**: American | **Cook**: 10 m

Ingredients
- 1/3 cup chopped Onions
- 1 tbsp Extra Virgin Olive Oil
- 1/2 cup shredded Cheddar Cheese
- 2 large Eggs (Whole)

Directions

1. Sauté white onions in 1 tablespoon virgin olive oil in a small skillet over medium heat until translucent and tender. Remove from pan and set aside.
2. Lightly beat eggs and add to the same skillet. Allow to form bubbles then carefully flip over. Spread cheese and onions over half the surface. Cook for 1 minute more, fold other side over onions and cheese. Cook 1 more minute.
3. Slide off skillet and on to plate. Season to taste with salt and freshly ground black pepper.

Nutritional Information
- Protein : 26.7g
- Fat : 41.8g
- Fiber : 0.9g
- Calories : 509

Cheddar Omelet With Sautéed Tomato And Zucchini

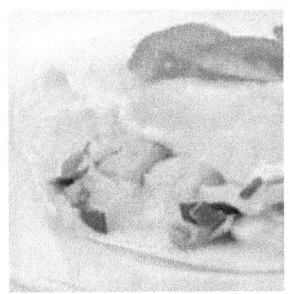

Servings: 1 | **Prep**: 5 m | **Style**: American | **Cook**: 10 m

Ingredients
- 1 tsp Olive Oil

- 1/2 cup chopped Zucchini
- 1/2 medium whole (2-3/5" dia) Red Tomatoes
- 2 large Eggs (Whole)
- 1/2 cup shredded Cheddar Cheese

Directions
1. Preheat a skillet with 1 teaspoon oil. Add chopped zucchini to pan and sauté until soft about 2-3 minutes. Add chopped tomatoes and heat through about 1 minute. Remove from skillet and set aside.
2. Pour slightly beaten eggs into the skillet and cook 2-3 minutes until large bubbles begin to form and bottom edge is set. Carefully lift one edge of omelet and flip over. Cook an additional 2 minutes.
3. Layer half of cheese onto half of the omelet then top with tomatoes and zucchini. Layer the second half of cheese over the vegetables then carefully flip over the other half of the omelet to sandwich in the cheese and veggies. Heat through until cheese begins to melt. Remove from heat to a serving plate and top with remaining vegetables.

Nutritional Information
- Protein : 27.3g
- Fat : 32.4g
- Fiber : 1.1g
- Calories :431

Cheddar Omelet With Sautéed Watercress

Servings: 1 | **Prep:** 5 m | **Style:** American | **Cook:** 8 m

Ingredients
- 1/2 cup chopped Watercress
- 2 large Eggs (Whole)
- 1/2 cup shredded Cheddar Cheese
- 1 tsp Extra Virgin Olive Oil

Directions
1. Heat oil in small nonstick skillet over medium-high heat. Add watercress and sauté for 1 minute until tender. Add salt and freshly ground black pepper to taste. Remove from skillet and set aside.
2. Add eggs to skillet and cook for 2 minutes on medium heat until underside is lightly browned. Flip and cook 1 more minute.
3. Add watercress to half of omelet and top with cheese. Fold over other half and cook for 1 more minute to melt cheese. Serve immediately.

Nutritional Information
- Protein : 26.5g
- Fat : 32.4g
- Fiber : 0.1g
- Calories :410

Cheddar Omelet With Swiss Chard And Onions

Servings: 1 | **Prep:** 5 m | **Style:** American | **Cook:** 8 m

Ingredients
- 1 tbsp Light Olive Oil
- 2 cups Swiss Chard
- 1/4 cup shredded Cheddar Cheese
- 2 large Eggs (Whole)
- 1/4 cup chopped Onions

Directions
1. Heat a nonstick skillet with 2 teaspoons oil over medium-high heat. Add white onions and sauté until tender. Quickly add chard and sauté until wilted. Squeeze as much water as possible from the chart by pressing it with the back of a spatula and draining. Remove from pan and set aside.
2. In same pan, add remaining teaspoon of oil and eggs and cook 2 -3 minutes till firm on one side. Flip and cook 1 more minute. To half of the omelet add onions and chard, top with cheese and fold over other half. Cook another 1 -2 minutes to melt cheese. Season to taste with salt and freshly ground black pepper and serve.

Nutritional Information
- Protein : 20.8g
- Fat : 32.5g
- Fiber : 1.8g
- Calories :404

Cheese And Spinach Omelet Topped With Avocado And Salsa

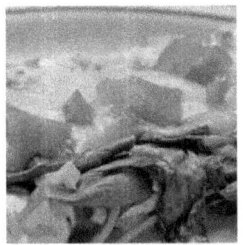

Servings: 1 | **Prep:** 5 m | **Style:** American | **Cook:** 10 m

Ingredients
- 1/2 fruit without skin and seed California Avocados
- 2 1/16 cups Baby Spinach
- 1 slice (1 oz) Monterey Jack Cheese
- 1 serving Salsa Cruda
- 2 large Eggs (Whole)
- 1 tbsp Extra Virgin Olive Oil

Directions

Use the Atkins recipe to make Salsa Cruda or use 2 tablespoons of no-sugar-added salsa.

1. Sauté spinach in a nonstick skillet with 1/2 tablespoon oil over medium high heat until wilted. Remove and set aside.
2. Lightly beat the eggs with salt and freshly ground black pepper.
3. Add 1/2 tablespoon oil to the same skillet used for the spinach then add the eggs. Cook for 3 minutes, flip over, and continue to cook on the other side for 2 minutes.

4. Add the cheese and sautéed spinach to half of the omelet. Flip other half over top. Cook an additional 1-2 minutes to melt cheese. Top with avocado and salsa.

Nutritional Information
- Protein : 21.9g
- Fat : 47.7g
- Fiber : 7.3g
- Calories :558

Cheese Baked Eggs

Servings: 1 | **Prep:** 5 m | **Style:** American | **Cook:** 10 m

Ingredients
- 1 tsp Unsalted Butter Stick
- 2 large Eggs (Whole)
- 2 tbsps Heavy Cream
- 2 tbsps Parmesan Cheese (Grated)

Directions
1. Melt butter and coat the inside of a small oven safe dish.
2. Combine the eggs and cream in a bowl and lightly beat.
3. Add parmesan cheese and freshly ground black pepper and salt to taste.
4. Bake at 375°F for 10 minutes or until set.

Nutritional Information
- Protein : 17.1g
- Fat : 27.3g
- Fiber : 0g
- Calories :324

Cheesy Bacon Cloud Muffin

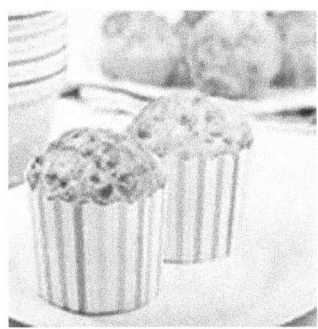

Servings: 1 | **Prep:** 1 m | **Style:** American | **Cook:** 1 m

Ingredients
- 1 oz Cream Cheese
- 1 large Egg
- 2 tbsps Vanilla Whey Protein
- 1/4 tsp Baking Powder (Sodium Aluminum Sulfate, Double Acting)
- 1 slice cooked Bacon (Cured, Pan-Fried, Cooked)
- 1 slice (1 oz) Cheddar Cheese

Directions
1. Place cream cheese in a microwave safe mug. Heat for 10-15 seconds (enough to warm the cream cheese but not to fully melt it).
2. Add the egg and whisk it with the cream cheese.
3. Add the whey protein powder (use a protein powder that has 1g NC or less per serving, one serving is about 1 oz) and baking powder; whisk to combine. Season with a pinch of salt and freshly ground black pepper.
4. Tear the cooked bacon into small pieces and cut the cheese into small pieces. Add them to the mixture, mixing to

combine. Heat the mug in the microwave for 1 min (microwave times vary so you may need to increase the time by 10-20 seconds if it does not cook through with 1 minute.) Remove muffin by turning over onto a plate. Run a knife around the inside of the mug to more easily release it.

Nutritional Information
- Protein : 28.9g
- Fat : 27.3g
- Fiber : 0g
- Calories :375

Chicken Chorizo And Cauliflower Saute With Cheese And Salsa

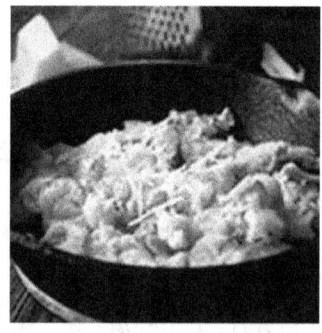

Servings: 1 | **Prep:** 5 m | **Style:** American | **Cook:** 15 m

Ingredients
- 1 cup Cauliflower
- 1 link Spicy Chorizo Chicken Sausage
- 1 slice (1 oz) Monterey Jack Cheese
- 2 tbsps Chunky Medium Salsa

Directions
1. Cut cauliflower into bite sized pieces and place in a medium non-stick skillet over medium-high heat. Add 2 Tbsp water and cook until water evaporates and cauliflower is crisp-tender (add more water as necessary to prevent burning). Once cauliflower is crisp-tender add the chorizo breaking it up in the pan with a spatula into bite sized pieces. Cook until sausage is cooked through. Remove from heat and place on a serving plate.
2. Top the cauliflower and chorizo with cheese, allowing it to melt. Serve once cheese has melted with 2 Tbsp fresh salsa.

Nutritional Information
- Protein : 23.9g
- Fat : 16.7g
- Fiber : 3.5g
- Calories :291

Chicken-Portobello Broilers

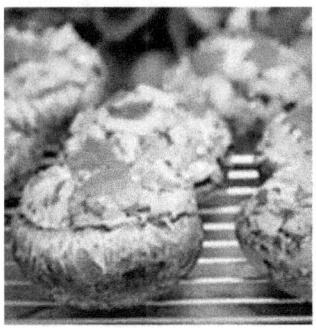

Servings: 6 | **Prep:** 10 m | **Style:** American | **Cook:** 20 m

Ingredients
- 2 tbsps Extra Virgin Olive Oil
- 8 oz raw (yield after cooking, bone removed) Chicken Breast
- 3 tbsps chopped Scallions or Spring Onions
- 4 large Eggs (Whole)
- 6 caps Portobello Mushroom Cap
- 1/4 tsp Salt
- 1/4 tsp Black Pepper
- 1/4 tsp Italian Seasoning
- 1/4 cup shredded Mozzarella Cheese (Whole Milk)

Directions
1. Preheat broiler.
2. Cut chicken breast in half lengthwise, then thinly slice crosswise.
3. Heat oil in a large nonstick skillet over medium heat. Add the chicken and green onion and cook 3 4 minutes until chicken is no longer pink. Add the eggs and cook until firm.
4. Meanwhile, place the mushroom caps, ribbed side up, on a foil-lined baking sheet. Sprinkle with salt, pepper and herbs and broil for about 7 minutes, turning once, until slightly soft and dark in color.
5. Remove mushroom caps from oven and spoon egg mixture into them. Optional: add freshly diced tomatoes or red bell pepper to increase your veggies for the day. Top with cheese and broil for 1 minute until melted.
6. Serve immediately.

Nutritional Information
- Protein : 15.1g
- Fat : 10.2g
- Fiber : 1.2g
- Calories :165

Chili Spiced "Tortilla" Wraps

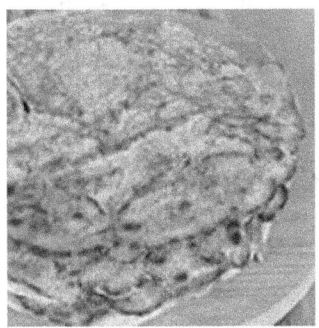

Servings: 4 | **Prep:** 5 m | **Style:** Mexican | **Cook:** 15 m

Ingredients
- 3 tbsps Organic High Fiber Coconut Flour
- 3/4 tsp Chili Powder
- 1/16 cup Organic 100% Whole Ground Golden Flaxseed Meal
- 1/8 tsp Salt
- 3 large Egg Whites
- 1/2 cup Coconut Milk Unsweetened
- 1 1/3 tbsps Light Olive Oil
- 1/2 tsp Xylitol

Directions
1. Combine the 3 tbsp coconut flour, chili powder, 1 tbsp flax meal, and salt in a small bowl. Set aside.
2. Whisk the egg whites, coconut milk, and sugar substitute. Add the flour mixture, mix to combine, then allow to sit for 5 minutes.
3. Heat a large skillet with 1 teaspoon of oil over medium-high heat. Using a 1/4 cup measure, pour batter into pan and spread out into a 5-inch tortilla shape. Allow to cook for 2-3 minutes, until golden brown underneath and set on the

top. Flip over and cook 1 additional minute. Repeat for remaining 3 tortillas.
4. Place cooked tortillas on a paper towel and a paper towel between each. Tortillas may be refrigerated for up to 1 week, store in an airtight container with the paper towels in between or freeze for up to 3 months.

Nutritional Information
- Protein : 3.8g
- Fat : 6.4g
- Fiber : 3g
- Calories :90

Chocolate And Strawberry Smoothie

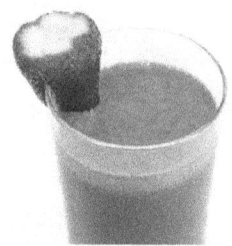

Servings: 1 | **Prep:** 5 m | **Style:** American

Ingredients
- 1/2 cup Frozen Strawberries
- 1 cup Coconut Milk Unsweetened
- 1 oz or 1 scoop Chocolate Whey Protein
- 2 tsps Cocoa Powder (Unsweetened)
- 1 pinch Stevia

Directions
1. For this recipe unsweetened coconut, almond or soy milk may be used.
2. Combine the frozen strawberries, milk of choice, protein powder, cocoa powder and stevia (to taste) in a blender. Blend until smooth.

Nutritional Information
- Protein : 20.9g
- Fat : 7.9g
- Fiber 4.3g
- Calories :193

Chocolate Cake Donuts

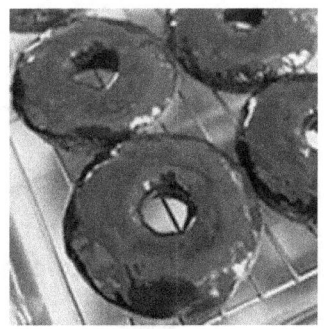

Servings: 6 | **Style**: American

Ingredients
- 7 tbsps Unsalted Butter Stick
- 3 large Eggs
- 1/8 cup Coconut Milk Unsweetened
- 5 tbsps Sucralose Based Sweetener (Sugar Substitute)
- 1 tsp Vanilla Extract

- 1/2 cup Almond Meal Flour
- 1/4 cup Cocoa Powder (Unsweetened)
- 2 tbsps Organic High Fiber Coconut Flour
- 1/2 tsp Cinnamon
- 1/4 tsp Baking Soda
- 1/4 tsp Baking Powder (Sodium Aluminum Sulfate, Double Acting)
- 1/4 tsp Salt
- 2 tbsps Heavy Cream
- 2 oz Sugar Free Chocolate Chips

Directions
1. Preheat oven to 350°F. Prepare a 6-well donut pan by spraying with oil and set it aside.
2. Melt 5 tbsp butter in a medium microwave safe bowl. Whisk in the eggs, coconut milk, granular sugar substitute, and vanilla until smooth.
3. In a small bowl whisk to combine the almond meal, cocoa power, coconut flour, cinnamon, baking soda, baking powder and salt. Add this mixture to the egg mixture whisking to combine in to a smooth thick batter. Pour into the wells of the donut pan and bake for 16-18 minutes until fragrant and set. Remove from oven to a cooling rack leaving them to sit in the pan for 10 minutes then remove from the pan and continue to cool on a wire rack.
4. Place the remaining 2 tbsp butter, heavy cream and sugar-free chocolate in a small microwave safe bowl that is slightly bigger than the width of the donuts. Melt at 30 second intervals (1 minute total) then whisk until smooth. Dip the tops of the donuts in the glaze and place back on the cooling rack to set the glaze (drizzle any remaining over the tops).. Enjoy immediately or refrigerate for up to 3 days in an airtight container. Serve at room temperature.

Nutritional Information
- Protein : 7.1g
- Fat : 26.4g
- Fiber 3.8g
- Calories :299

Chocolate Cloud Muffin

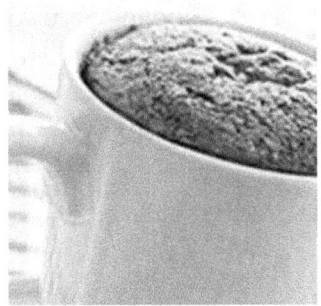

Servings: 1 | **Prep**: 1 m | **Style**: American | **Cook:** 1 m

Ingredients
- 1 oz Cream Cheese
- 1 large Egg
- 1 tbsp Vegetable Oil
- 2 tbsps Vanilla Whey Protein
- 2 tsps Cocoa Powder (Unsweetened)
- 2 tsps Xylitol
- 1/4 tsp Baking Powder (Sodium Aluminum Sulfate, Double Acting)
- 1/2 tsp Cinnamon
- 1/8 tsp Salt
- 1 packet 100% Natural Stevia Sweetener

Directions
1. Place cream cheese in a microwave safe mug. Heat for 10-15 seconds (enough to warm the cream cheese but not to fully melt it).
2. Add the egg and oil whisking them into the cream cheese.
3. In a small bowl mix to combine the whey protein powder, cocoa powder, xylitol, baking powder, cinnamon, and a pinch of salt and stevia (a whole packet may be too much or just right for your taste - you may need to experiment).
4. Add the chocolate mixture to the cream cheese mixture in the cup; stir to combine. (Be sure to us a protein powder that has 1g NC or less per serving, one serving is about 1 oz).
5. Heat the mug in the microwave for 1 min (microwave times vary so you may need to increase the time by 10-20 seconds if it does not cook through with 1 minute.) Remove muffin by turning over onto a plate. Run a knife around the inside of the mug to more easily release it.

Nutritional Information
- Protein : 19.7g
- Fat : 29g
- Fiber : 9.8g
- Calories :371

Chocolate Hazelnut Smoothie

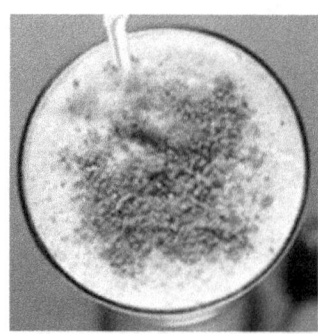

Servings: 2 | **Prep:** 3 m | **Style:** American

Ingredients
- 2 scoops Chocolate Whey Protein
- 1 tbsp Heavy Cream
- 12 tsps Sugar Free Hazelnut Syrup

Directions
1. Place protein mix, cream and syrup in a blender with about 1/2 cup of ice; blend until smooth.
2. Pour into 2 glasses. Sprinkle with cinnamon, if desired.

Nutritional Information
- Protein : 23.2g
- Fat : 22.2g
- Fiber : 0g
- Calories :297

Chocolate Peanut Butter Smoothie

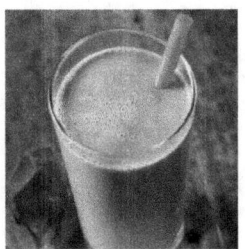

Servings: 1 | **Prep:** 5 m | **Style:** American | **Cook:** 1 m

Ingredients

- 1 cup Coconut Milk Unsweetened
- 2 tbsps Natural Creamy Peanut Butter 1/3 Less Sodium & Sugar
- 1 tbsp Cocoa Powder (Unsweetened)
- 1 scoop Chocolate Whey Protein
- 1/4 tsp Cinnamon
- 1 pinch Stevia
- 1/16 tsp Salt

Directions
1. For this recipe unsweetened coconut, almond or soy milk may be used.
2. Combine the ice, milk of choice, peanut butter, protein powder, cocoa powder, cocoa powder, stevia and salt (to taste) in a blender. Blend until smooth.

Nutritional Information
- Protein : 29g
- Fat : 24.2g
- Fiber : 5.6g
- Calories :361

Chorizo, Green Chili And Tomato Frittata

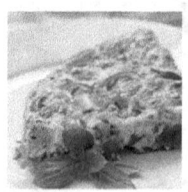

Servings: 6 | **Prep:** 10 m | **Style:** American | **Cook:** 15 m

Ingredients
- 6 oz Pork and Beef Chorizo
- 12 large Eggs (Whole)
- 8 oz Green Chili Peppers (Canned)
- 2/3 cup chopped or sliced Red Tomatoes
- 2 oz Cheddar Cheese

Directions
1. Preheat broiler.
2. In a large oven-proof skillet, sauté the chorizo, breaking it up into bite-sized pieces over medium-high heat until cooked through; about 5 minutes. Drain off excess fat and leave in the pan.
3. Add lightly beaten eggs, green chilies, tomatoes and cheese to the chorizo. Cook over medium-high heat for 4-5 minutes then place pan under the broiler for 3-4 minutes until light and slightly puffed. Serve immediately.

Nutritional Information
- Protein : 24.3g
- Fat : 26.7g
- Fiber : 1.5g
- Calories :362

Cinnamon Buns

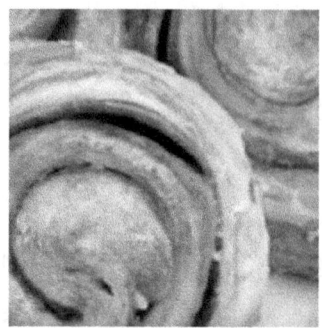

Servings: 12 | **Prep:** 20 m | **Style:** American | **Cook:** 35 m

Ingredients
- 1 1/2 tsps Baking Powder (Straight Phosphate, Double Acting)
- 1/2 tsp Salt
- 1/2 cup Unsalted Butter Stick
- 2 large Egg Yolks
- 1 1/2 cups Tap Water
- 1 tsp Cinnamon
- 6 tbsps Sucralose Based Sweetener (Sugar Substitute)
- 1/2 cup chopped Pecans
- 1 1/2 oz Dried Currants
- 1 tbsp Heavy Cream
- 6 servings All Purpose Low-Carb Baking Mix
- 5 1/4 tbsps Sugar Free Brown Sugar Cinnamon Syrup

Directions

Use the Atkins recipe to make All Purpose Low-Carb Baking Mix for this recipe.

1. In a large bowl mix baking mix (you will need 2 cups of the above recipe), baking powder, salt, water, 4 tablespoons butter, 4 tablespoons sugar substitute and 1 egg yolk until smooth. Cover lightly with plastic wrap and let rise one hour. Stretch dough out to a rectangle measuring 10x15 inches, long side facing towards you.
2. For filling: mix 4 tablespoons butter, 2 tablespoons sugar substitute and cinnamon. Brush mixture over dough, leaving a ½ border at the bottom. Sprinkle dough evenly with nuts and currants. Roll dough up lengthwise from the top, stretching it as you go along. Pinch dough tightly to seal roll and pat to even out shape if necessary. Cut dough roll in half, then halve each half, then cut each quarter into thirds (you will have 12 even slices). Arrange slices on a nonstick baking sheet, lightly cover with plastic wrap and let rise 45 minutes. Heat oven to 375°F.
3. Mix 1 egg yolk and cream. Brush dough slices with mixture. Bake 30 to 35 minutes until lightly browned. Cool buns five minutes then brush with sugar-free cinnamon syrup. Serve warm or at room temperature.

Nutritional Information
- Protein : 16.7g
- Fat : 14.3g
- Fiber : 2.3g
- Calories :218

Cinnamon Churritos

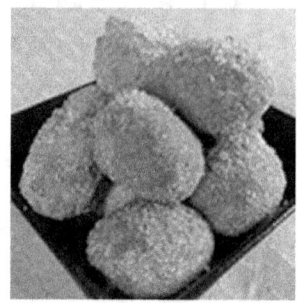

Servings: 8 | **Prep:** 10 m | **Style:** American | **Cook:** 10 m

Ingredients
- 1/2 cup Blanched Almond Flour
- 2 tbsps Organic High Fiber Coconut Flour
- 1/4 tsp Baking Powder (Straight Phosphate, Double Acting)
- 2 tsps Cinnamon
- 1/8 tsp Salt
- 1/2 cup Coconut Milk Unsweetened
- 1 tbsp Unsalted Butter Stick
- 3 tbsps Xylitol
- 1 large Egg (Whole)

Directions

These are acceptable only for the fast track of Phase 1 because they contain almonds.

1. Prepare a large skillet or deep fat fryer with 2-3 inches of oil. Heat to 350°F. In a small bowl combine the almond flour, coconut flour, baking powder, 1 teaspoon cinnamon and salt. Mix thoroughly and set aside.

2. In a small sauce pan bring the coconut milk, butter and 1 tablespoon xylitol to a boil. Remove from heat and add the flour mixture stirring until very thick and it forms a ball. Allow to cool for 5 minutes.
3. Once cool add 1 egg and mix until a very thick paste forms, about 1 minute. Drop by tablespoons 4-8 at a time into the fryer and fry until golden brown and crisp on the outside; about 3-4 minutes; rotating halfway through. Repeat until all of batter is used. It should make about 16 balls. Set aside on a paper towel once cooked.
4. In a blender pulse the remaining 2 tablespoons of xylitol with 1 teaspoon of cinnamon 1-2 times, until xylitol granules are a little smaller. When each batch is finished roll in the xylitol-cinnamon mixture until evenly coated and set on a serving platter. Enjoy immediately or they may be kept at room temperature for 1 day. May also freeze for 3 months or refrigerate for up to 1 week. 2 balls per serving.

Nutritional Information
- Protein : 2.6g
- Fat : 6.1g
- Fiber : 6.3g
- Calories :85

Cinnamon Crumb Coffee Cake

Servings: 12 | **Prep:** 30 m | **Style:** American | **Cook:** 40 m

Ingredients
- 3/4 cup 100% Stone Ground Whole Wheat Pastry Flour
- 1/2 cup Whole Wheat Flour
- 1 tsp Baking Powder (Straight Phosphate, Double Acting)
- 1 tsp Baking Soda

- 1/2 tsp Salt
- 2 large Eggs (Whole)
- 1 tsp Vanilla Extract
- 1 cup Sour Cream (Cultured)
- 1 1/4 cups Unsalted Butter Stick
- 2 cups Sucralose Based Sweetener (Sugar Substitute)
- 1/2 cup, dry, yield Oatmeal
- 3/4 cup Whole Grain Soy Flour
- 1 1/2 cup halves Pecan Nuts
- 2 tsps Cinnamon

Directions
1. Preheat oven to 350°F. Grease a 9x13 inch baking pan and set aside.
2. For cake: In a medium bowl, whisk together pastry flour, soy flour, whole-wheat flour, baking powder, baking soda and salt. In a large liquid measuring cup whisk eggs, vanilla and sour cream until well combined.
3. In a large bowl, with an electric mixer on medium speed, beat 1/2 cup butter and 1 cup sugar substitute until smooth and fluffy, about 4 minutes. Alternately add the flour mixture and egg mixture to the butter, beginning and ending with the flour mixture.
4. For topping: In a blender, pulse oats, 1 cup sugar substitute, pecans, 3/4 cup butter and cinnamon until texture resembles a coarse meal.
5. To assemble cake: Spread two-thirds of the batter into the prepared pan. Sprinkle half the topping over batter and lightly swirl with a knife to create pockets of topping within the batter.
6. Spoon remaining batter over topping, and sprinkle evenly with remaining topping. Bake until a knife inserted in the center comes out clean, about 40 minutes. Cool cake in pan set over a wire rack. Serve warm or at room temperature. Makes 12 servings.

Nutritional Information
- Protein : 6.4g
- Fat : 33.6g
- Fiber : 3.9g
- Calories :397

Cinnamon Mini Muffins

Servings: 24 | **Prep:** 15 m | **Style:** American | **Cook:** 20 m

Ingredients
- 1/2 cup Blanched & Slivered Almonds
- 1/2 cup dry Whole Grain Soy Flour
- 1 tbsp Cinnamon
- 1/4 tsp Salt
- 1/2 tsp Baking Powder (Straight Phosphate, Double Acting)
- 1/2 cup Unsalted Butter Stick
- 3 large Eggs (Whole)
- 2 tsps Vanilla Extract
- 3/4 cup Sucralose Based Sweetener (Sugar Substitute)

Directions
1. Heat oven to 350°F. Spray mini-muffin tins with cooking spray.
2. Pulse almonds in bowl of food processor and 1 tablespoon soy flour until almonds are finely ground (the soy flour will prevent over processing of almonds). Add remaining soy flour, cinnamon, salt and baking powder; pulse to combine.
3. With an electric mixer on medium speed, beat butter and sugar substitute in until fluffy, 3 to 4 minutes. Beat in vanilla extract. Add eggs, one at a time, beating well after each addition. Fold in almond mixture with a spatula.

4. Fill muffin tins 2/3 full with batter. Bake 20 minutes or until set in middle. Transfer to wire rack for 5 minutes to cool. Turn out muffins on to rack to cool completely.

Nutritional Information
- Protein : 2.1g
- Fat : 6.3g
- Fiber : 0.7g
- Calories :73

Coconut-Vanilla Shake

Servings: 4 | **Prep:** 5 m | **Style:** American

Ingredients
- 1 14 oz can Coconut Cream
- 2 scoops Vanilla Whey Protein
- 1/2 tsp Vanilla Extract

Directions
1. Place coconut cream, protein powder, vanilla and 2 cups of ice cubes in a blender and pulse until smooth and creamy.

Nutritional Information
- Protein : 21.8g
- Fat : 23.9g
- Fiber : 0.6g
- Calories :310

Corned Beef Hash

Servings: 4 | **Prep:** 5 m | **Style:** Other | **Cook:** 20 m

Ingredients
- 16 oz Corned Beef Brisket (Cured)
- 2 cups Turnips (with Salt, Frozen, Drained, Cooked, Boiled)
- 1/2 cup chopped Onions
- 1/2 cup Heavy Cream
- 3 tbsps Canola Vegetable Oil

Directions

For this recipe canned or frozen turnips may be substituted for freshly cooked cubed turnips.

1. Toss cubed beef and turnips together in a bowl. Add onion and heavy cream and stir to combine.
2. Heat oil in a heavy nonstick skillet over medium-low heat 1 minute. Add beef-turnip mixture and cook until a crust forms, about 10 minutes.
3. Turn hash and brown other side, about 10 minutes more. Serve with a poached egg, if desired (adds .4g NC to each serving).

Nutritional Information
- Protein : 22g
- Fat : 43.2g
- Fiber : 1.9g
- Calories :506

Creamy Scrambled Eggs With Dill And Smoked Salmon

Servings: 4 | **Prep:** 10 m | **Style:** American | **Cook:** 15 m

Ingredients
- 4 medium (4-1/8" long) Scallions or Spring Onions
- 3 tbsps Heavy Cream
- 1/2 tsp Salt
- 8 large Eggs (Whole)
- 4 tbsps Unsalted Butter Stick
- 6 oz Smoked Chinook Salmon (Lox)
- 1 tbsp Dill (Dried)

Directions
1. In a large bowl, beat eggs, cream, dill and salt.
2. Melt butter in a large skillet over medium heat. Add scallions; cook 8 minutes until softened. Pour in egg mixture; cook 3 4 minutes, stirring occasionally, until almost set.
3. Mix in salmon, cook 1 minute more or until eggs reach desired doneness.
4. Transfer to warmed plates.

Nutritional Information
- Protein : 20.4g
- Fat : 26.5g
- Fiber : 0.4g
- Calories :335

Crunchy Tropical Berry And Almond Breakfast Parfait

Servings: 4 | **Prep:** 20 m | **Style:** American | **Cook:** 15 m

Ingredients
- 1/2 cup Heavy Cream
- 1 1/2 tsps Sucralose Based Sweetener (Sugar Substitute)

- 1/4 tsp Coconut Extract
- 1/2 cup 2% Plain Greek Yogurt
- 1 cup Red Raspberries
- 1 cup Blueberries
- 1/2 cup Dried Coconut
- 4 servings Sweet and Salty Almonds

Directions

Use the Atkins recipe to make Sweet and Salty Almonds for this recipe. You will need 1/2 cup.

1. Combine cream, 1/2 teaspoon sugar substitute, and coconut (or vanilla) extract in a medium bowl; whip with an electric mixer on medium speed until stiff peaks form. Fold in the yogurt.
2. Puree raspberries and remaining sugar substitute in a blender until smooth.
3. Using 4 parfait glasses, alternate layers of whipped cream, raspberry puree, blueberries, nuts, and coconut, making two layers of each. Serve right away.

Nutritional Information
- Protein : 6.9g
- Fat : 28.3g
- Fiber : 6g
- Calories :341

Crustless Broccoli Quiche

Servings: 6 | **Prep:** 15 m | **Style:** American | **Cook:** 60 m

Ingredients

- 1 tsp Extra Virgin Olive Oil
- 1 cup Half and Half Cream
- 1 cup shredded Cheddar Cheese
- 1/2 cup Tap Water
- 1/4 tsp Thyme
- 1/4 tsp leaf Oregano
- 1/2 tsp Salt
- 4 large Eggs (Whole)
- 1/4 tsp Black Pepper
- 1/4 tsp Rosemary (Dried)
- 1 lb Broccoli Flower Clusters
- 1/2 small Onion

Directions
1. Preheat oven to 375°F.
2. Brush a 9- or 10-inch pie plate with virgin olive oil.
3. Heat oil in a small skillet over medium-high heat. Add white onion and cook until softened, about 3 minutes. Transfer to a medium bowl; let cool.
4. Add eggs to onion and lightly beat. Whisk in dairy beverage, 1/2 cup cheese, water, thyme, oregano, salt, pepper and rosemary to blend.
5. Cover bottom of pie plate with broccoli. Pour egg mixture over it and sprinkle with remaining 1/2 cup cheese.
6. Bake until a knife inserted in middle comes out clean and quiche is golden brown, 50 to 60 minutes. Alternatively, these may be baked in a greased muffin tin for 15-20 minutes until fully set. They make an easy on-the-go meal or snack.

Nutritional Information
- Protein : 12g
- Fat : 18g
- Fiber : 2.1g

- Calories :236

Crustless Pumpkin And Ham Quiche

Servings: 8 | **Prep:** 10 m | **Style:** American | **Cook:** 30 m

Ingredients
- 1 medium (2-1/2" dia) Onions
- 2 tbsps Unsalted Butter Stick
- 4 large Eggs
- 1/2 cup Heavy Cream
- 1 cup mashed Cooked Pumpkin
- 1/2 cup Ham (Whole, Cured, Roasted)
- 1 tbsp Parsley
- 1 cup shredded Gruyere Cheese
- 1/8 tsp Red or Cayenne Pepper

Directions
1. Preheat oven to 350°F. Prepare a pie plate with oil. Set aside.
2. In a small skillet saute the dice onion in the butter until soft; about 6 minutes.
3. In a large bowl whisk together the eggs and cream. Add the pumpkin, diced ham, sauteed onion, chopped parsley and cheese. Season with salt and freshly ground black pepper (about 1/4 tsp each) and the cayenne pepper (optional).
4. Pour into prepared pie plate and bake for 30-35 minutes until puffed and set in the center. Transfer to a wire rack to cool. Enjoy warm or cold.

Nutritional Information
- Protein : 9.9g
- Fat : 17.3g

- Fiber : 1.1g
- Calories :211

Crustless Spinach Quiche

Servings: 4 | **Prep:** 20 m | **Style:** American | **Cook:** 30 m

Ingredients
- 2 tsps Canola Vegetable Oil
- 6 1/2 oz Frozen Chopped Spinach
- 1/2 cup chopped Scallions or Spring Onions
- 1 cup Heavy Cream
- 1 cup shredded Muenster Cheese
- 1/4 tsp Salt
- 4 large Eggs (Whole)
- 1/8 tsp Nutmeg (Ground)
- 1/4 tsp Black Pepper

Directions
1. Preheat oven to 350°F (175°C). Lightly grease a 9 inch pie pan.
2. Heat oil in a large skillet over medium-high heat. Add onions and cook, stirring occasionally, until onions are soft. Stir in spinach and continue cooking until excess moisture has evaporated.
3. In a large bowl, combine eggs, cream, cheese, salt, 1/8 tsp nutmeg and pepper. Add spinach mixture and stir to blend. Pour into prepared pie pan.
4. Bake in preheated oven until eggs have set, about 30 minutes. Let cool for 10 minutes before serving.

Nutritional Information
- Protein : 15.2g

- Fat : 37.6g
- Fiber : 1.5g
- Calories :417

Double-Chocolate Express Smoothie

Servings: 1 | **Prep:** 5 m | **Style:** American | **Cook:** 30 m

Ingredients
- 1/2 cup Tap Water
- 3 tbsps Half and Half Cream
- 1 1/2 oz or 1 scoops Chocolate Whey Protein
- 1 tbsp Cocoa Powder (Unsweetened)
- 3/4 tsp rounded Coffee (Instant Powder, Decaffeinated)

Directions
1. Combine the water, half-and-half, protein powder, cocoa and espresso powders in a blender; blend until smooth. With the machine running, add 3-4 ice cubes, one at a time, and blend until smooth.
2. Pour into a tall glass, and garnish with a dusting of cocoa powder or drizzle with sugar-free chocolate syrup, if desired. Serve immediately.

Nutritional Information
- Protein : 35.5g
- Fat : 5.9g
- Fiber : 1.8g
- Calories :209

Dutch Baby Baked Pancake

Servings: 6 | **Prep:** 15 m | **Style:** American | **Cook:** 15 m

Ingredients
- 3 tbsps Unsalted Butter Stick
- 1/2 tsp Cinnamon
- 1/4 cup dry Whole Grain Soy Flour
- 1/4 tsp Salt
- 1/2 cup Heavy Cream
- 3 large Eggs (Whole)
- 5 tbsps Sucralose Based Sweetener (Sugar Substitute)
- 1/2 cup 100% Stone Ground Whole Wheat Pastry Flour
- 2 medium (2-3/4" dia) (approx 3 per lb) Apples

Directions
1. Heat oven to 425°F. Place 2 tablespoons of the butter in a 12-inch nonstick ovenproof skillet; set aside.
2. Whisk eggs, pastry flour, soy flour, salt, cream, 3 tablespoons of the sugar substitute and ¼ cup water together until smooth. Place skillet in oven until butter melts. Pour batter into skillet. Bake 15 minutes.
3. While pancake is baking, melt remaining tablespoon of butter in a medium skillet over medium heat. Add remaining 2 tablespoons sugar substitute, cinnamon and ¼ cup water. Bring to a boil; add apples. Cook 15 minutes over a low heat, stirring occasionally, until apples are tender and most of the liquid has evaporated.
4. After removing pancake from the oven, spoon apples into the center. Serve immediately.

Nutritional Information
- Protein : 5.8g
- Fat : 16.4g
- Fiber : 3g
- Calories :238

Eggs And Spinach

Servings: 1 | **Prep:** 5 m | **Style:** American | **Cook:** 5 m

Ingredients
- 1 tbsp Extra Virgin Olive Oil
- 2 1/16 cups Baby Spinach
- 2 large Eggs (Whole)

Directions
1. Add oil to a small skillet over medium heat. Add spinach and sauté until wilted.
2. Add eggs to skillet and scramble together until eggs are set.
3. Season to taste with salt and freshly ground black pepper before serving.

Nutritional Information
- Protein : 13.7g
- Fat : 13.9g
- Fiber : 1.3g
- Calories :194

Eggs Scrambled With Asparagus, Bacon And Swiss Cheese

Servings: 1 | **Prep:** 5 m | **Style:** American | **Cook:** 10 m

Ingredients
- 2 medium slice (yield after cooking) Bacon
- 1 large Egg (Whole)

- 1 oz Swiss Cheese
- 2 spear medium (5-1/4" to 7" long) Asparagus

Directions
1. Cook bacon in a small skillet over medium high heat. Reserve some of the bacon fat in the skillet and discard the rest or save for another use. Chop bacon into small pieces and set aside.
2. Cook asparagus in skillet with reserved bacon grease until tender, about 3 minutes. Remove and cut into bite-size pieces.
3. Add eggs, bacon, cheese and asparagus back to pan and scramble together until egg is cooked and cheese is melted, about 3 minutes. Or omit the cheese and instead sprinkle over the eggs after they are cooked.
4. Season to taste with salt and freshly ground black pepper.

Nutritional Information
- Protein : 19.7g
- Fat : 32.8g
- Fiber : 0.8g
- Calories :393

Eggs Scrambled With Avocado, Onions And Tomato

Servings: 1 | **Prep:** 5 m | **Style:** American | **Cook:** 10 m

Ingredients
- 1/2 fruit without skin and seed California Avocados
- 2 large Eggs (Whole)
- 1 small whole (2-2/5" dia) Red Tomato
- 2 tbsps chopped Onions

- 1 tsp Extra Virgin Olive Oil

Directions
1. Heat oil in a nonstick skillet over medium-high heat.
2. Sauté white onions in skillet until translucent.
3. Add eggs, avocado and tomatoes and scramble together until eggs are set.
4. Season to taste with salt and freshly ground black pepper and serve immediately.

Nutritional Information
- Protein : 14.4g
- Fat : 24.3g
- Fiber : 6.1g
- Calories :318

Eggs Scrambled With Cheddar And Swiss Chard

Servings: 1 | **Prep:** 5 m | **Style:** American | **Cook:** 8 m

Ingredients
- 2 cups Swiss Chard
- 2 large Eggs (Whole)
- 1/4 cup shredded Cheddar Cheese
- 1 tsp Extra Virgin Olive Oil

Directions

1. In a small skillet or sauté pan with 1 teaspoon of canola oil over medium heat, sauté Swiss chard just until decreased in volume and tender, 2 3 minutes.
2. Add eggs to skillet with chard. Using a spatula, mix to combine and scramble until eggs are set.
3. Top with cheese (or add it with the eggs and cook together) and serve immediately.

Nutritional Information
- Protein : 20.3g
- Fat : 23.2g
- Fiber : 1.2g
- Calories :308

Eggs Scrambled With Cheddar, Swiss Chard And Canadian Bacon

Servings: 1 | **Prep:** 5 m | **Style:** American | **Cook:** 8 m

Ingredients
- 2 large Eggs (Whole)
- 2 cups Swiss Chard
- 1/4 cup shredded Cheddar Cheese
- 1 tbsp Extra Virgin Olive Oil
- 2 oz Canadian-Style Bacon (Cured)

Directions
1. Sauté Swiss chard in 1 tsp oil until decreased in volume and tender.
2. Beat eggs slightly and add to pan with Swiss chard. Using a spatula mix to combine and cook till eggs are set.
3. Add shredded Cheddar cheese and Canadian bacon to top or it may be added in with the eggs and cooked all together.

Nutritional Information
- Protein : 32.6g
- Fat : 27.6g
- Fiber : 1.2g
- Calories :400

Eggs Scrambled With Feta And Spinach

Servings: 1 | **Prep:** 5 m | **Style:** American | **Cook:** 5 m

Ingredients
- 1 tbsp Canola Vegetable Oil
- 2 1/16 cups Baby Spinach
- 2 large Eggs (Whole)
- 1/2 oz Feta Cheese

Directions
1. In a small non-stick skillet, wilt spinach with 1 tablespoon of water over medium heat.
2. Add lightly beaten eggs and cheese and cook until set.
3. Season with salt and freshly ground black pepper and serve immediately.

Nutritional Information
- Protein : 16.9g
- Fat : 27.7g
- Fiber : 1.3g
- Calories :330

Eggs Scrambled With Sautéed Mushrooms And Zucchini

Servings: 1 | **Prep:** 5 m | **Style:** American | **Cook:** 10 m

Ingredients
- 1/2 cup Mushroom Pieces and Stems
- 1/2 cup chopped Zucchini
- 1 tbsp Extra Virgin Olive Oil
- 2 large Eggs (Whole)

Directions
1. Dice zucchini.
2. In a small non-stick skillet, saute the zucchini and mushrooms in the olive oil until softened, about 5 minutes. Season with salt and freshly ground black pepper.
3. Pour in slightly beaten eggs and scramble togther with the vegetables until eggs are set.

Nutritional Information
- Protein : 13.8g
- Fat : 23.3g
- Fiber : 0.9g
- Calories :278

Eggs Scrambled With Sautéed Onions And Cheddar Cheese

Servings: 1 | **Prep:** 5 m | **Style:** American | **Cook:** 10 m

Ingredients
- 1 tsp Canola Vegetable Oil
- 1/4 cup shredded Cheddar Cheese
- 1/4 cup chopped Onions
- 2 large Eggs (Whole)

Directions
1. Heat oil in a skillet over medium-high heat. Add white onions and sauté for 3 minutes until tender.
2. Add eggs and cheese and scramble together, cooking until eggs are set.
3. Season with salt and freshly ground pepper. Serve immediately.

Nutritional Information
- Protein : 19.5g
- Fat : 23.1g
- Fiber : 0.7g
- Calories :311

Eggs Scrambled With Zucchini, Cheddar And Sour Cream

Servings: 1 | **Prep:** 10 m | **Style:** American | **Cook:** 10 m

Ingredients
- 2 tbsps Sour Cream (Cultured)
- 1/2 cup chopped Zucchini
- 2 large Eggs (Whole)
- 1 tsp Extra Virgin Olive Oil
- 1/4 cup shredded Cheddar Cheese

Directions
1. Lightly beat together eggs and sour cream. Set aside.
2. Heat a skillet over medium-high heat. Lightly sauté zucchini in oil for 2 minutes.

3. Add egg-sour cream mixture and cheese to the skillet and scramble together until thoroughly cooked.

Nutritional Information
- Protein : 20.3g
- Fat : 28g
- Fiber : 0.6g
- Calories :351

Eggs With Avocado And Salsa With Cantaloupe And Sausage

Servings: 1 | **Prep:** 5 m | **Style:** American | **Cook:** 10 m

Ingredients
- 2 large Eggs (Whole)
- 1 oz Salsa
- 1 wedge large (1/8 large melon) Cantaloupe Melons
- 4 oz Turkey Sausage
- 1/2 fruit without skin and seed California Avocados

Directions
1. Fry eggs (scramble or poach if desired instead).
2. Layer avocado then eggs then top with salsa.
3. Heat sausage in a medium skillet over high heat for about 5 minutes, until cooked through and nicely browned on all sides.
4. Cut cantaloupe and serve with turkey sausage and eggs.

Nutritional Information
- Protein : 35.9g
- Fat : 28.9g

- Fiber : 5.9g
- Calories :474

Eggs With Avocado And Salsa

Servings: 1 | **Prep:** 5 m | **Style:** American | **Cook:** 5 m

Ingredients
- 1/2 fruit without skin and seed California Avocados
- 1 oz Salsa
- 2 large Eggs (Whole)

Directions
1. Fry eggs in 1 teaspoon of virgin olive oil in a small skillet over medium high heat until desired doneness. Flip, if desired.
2. Season with salt and freshly ground black pepper.
3. Spread the avocado slices on a plate, top with eggs and then salsa.

Nutritional Information
- Protein : 14.3g
- Fat : 20.1g
- Fiber : 5g
- Calories :267

Eggs With Avocado And Tomato

Servings: 1 | **Prep:** 5 m | **Style:** American | **Cook:** 10 m

Ingredients
- 2 large Eggs (Whole)
- 1/2 medium whole (2-3/5" dia) Red Tomatoes

- 1/2 fruit without skin and seed California Avocados

Directions
1. Cook egg any way desired.
2. Slice tomato and avocado.
3. Layer tomato, avocado, and eggs. Sprinkle with paprika if desired

Nutritional Information
- Protein : 13.8 g
- Fat : 19.5g
- Fiber : 5.1g
- Calories :266

Eggs With Avocado, Salsa And Turkey Bacon

Servings: 1 | **Prep:** 5 m | **Style:** American | **Cook:** 15 m

Ingredients
- 1 oz Salsa
- 2 oz cooked Turkey Bacon
- 1/2 fruit without skin and seed California Avocados
- 2 large Eggs (Whole)

Directions
1. Slice avocado.
2. Fry eggs (scramble or poach if desired instead).
3. Cook turkey bacon slices on frying pan until crispy.
4. Layer avocado, eggs then bacon and top with salsa.

Nutritional Information
- Protein : 22.3 g

- Fat : 31g
- Fiber : 5g
- Calories :406

Eggs With Avocado, Tomato And Sausage

Servings: 1 | **Prep:** 5 m | **Style:** American | **Cook:** 8 m

Ingredients
- 1/2 avocado, ns as to florida or californium Avocados
- 1/2 medium whole (2-3/5" dia) Red Tomatoes
- 2 large Eggs (Whole)
- 3 oz raw (yield after cooking) Pork Sausage Patty or Link

Directions
1. Prepare eggs as desired by poaching, frying, scrambling or as an omelet.
2. Form non-link sausage into a patty and cook over medium-high heat in a skillet, or if linked cook until no longer pink in the center; about 5 minutes. Cook alone or with the eggs.
3. Top eggs with avocado and tomato (or fill omelet).
4. Serve with sausage.

Nutritional Information
- Protein : 27.2 g
- Fat : 42.6g
- Fiber : 5.1g
- Calories :528

Eggs With Cheddar, Asparagus, Salsa And Sour Cream

Servings: 1 | **Prep:** 5 m | **Style:** American | **Cook:** 10 m

Ingredients
- 4 spear medium (5-1/4" to 7" long) Asparagus
- 2 large Eggs (Whole)
- 1/4 cup shredded Cheddar Cheese
- 1/2 oz Salsa
- 1 tbsp Sour Cream (Cultured)

Directions
1. Steam asparagus in skillet for 3 minutes with 2 Tbsp water. Drain and chop.
2. Beat eggs and add to skillet with 1 tsp oil over medium heat. Add asparagus and cheddar and scramble with eggs till set.
3. Top with salsa and sour cream.

Nutritional Information
- Protein : 27.21.2 g
- Fat : 20.8g
- Fiber : 51.8g
- Calories :298

Farmers Breakfast Soup

Servings: 4 | **Prep:** 10 m | **Style:** American | **Cook:** 45 m

Ingredients
- 1/2 cup chopped Onions
- 2 medium slice (yield after cooking) Bacon
- 8 oz Turkey Sausage
- 4 oz Ground Beef (80% Lean / 20% Fat)
- 2/3 cup High Protein TVP (Textured Vegetable Protein)

- 1/2 cup chopped Celery
- 1/2 cup chopped Carrots
- 4 cups Chicken Broth, Bouillon or Consomme
- 1/4 tsp Black Pepper

Directions
1. In a large nonstick skillet, over medium heat, cook the bacon until it begins to brown. Add the sausage and beef to brown, breaking up the meat into small bits with a spatula or spoon (about 7 minutes).
2. Stir in the TVP and vegetables. Cook 5 minutes until vegetables begin to soften.
3. Add remaining ingredients and simmer for 20 minutes, skimming off excess fat from the surface of the liquid.
4. Season with salt and pepper to taste.

Nutritional Information
- Protein : 26.8 g
- Fat : 14.4g
- Fiber : 3.6g
- Calories :277

Fennel, Carrot Hash And Turkey Hash

Servings: 6 | **Prep:** 10 m | **Style:** American | **Cook:** 20 m

Ingredients
- 2 tbsps Canola Vegetable Oil
- 6 oz Fennel Bulk
- 1/2 cup chopped Carrots
- 1/4 cup Freshly Squeezed Orange Juice
- 1 tbsp Orange Peel
- 1/4 tsp Fennel Seed

- 1 tbsp Tamari Soybean Sauce
- 1/2 cup chopped Scallions or Spring Onions
- 12 oz Turkey Breast Meat (Fryer-Roasters, Cooked, Roasted)

Directions

Top each serving with a poached egg, if desired

1. In a large skillet over medium heat, heat oil; add the fennel and carrot and sauté for about 3 minutes.
2. Add orange juice and zest. Simmer until liquid is almost absorbed, about 4 minutes.
3. Stir in fennel seeds, tamari, scallions and turkey. Cook for another 6 minutes until the turkey is heated through.

Nutritional Information
- Protein : 17.8 g
- Fat : 5.2g
- Fiber : 1.5g
- Calories :139

Feta And Red Bell Pepper Omelet

Servings: 1 | **Prep:** 5 m | **Style:** American | **Cook:** 10 m

Ingredients
- 1 tsp Extra Virgin Olive Oil
- 1/2 cup chopped Sweet Red Peppers
- 2 large Eggs (Whole)
- 2 oz Feta Cheese

Directions

1. Heat oil in a nonstick skillet over medium-high heat. Add bell pepper and sauté until tender. Remove from pan and set aside.
2. Add eggs to pan and cook 2 minutes till underside is golden. Using a spatular and tilting the skillet, flip over. Place the sautéed bell pepper topped with cheese on half the eggs.
3. Gently flip the other half over the mixture and cook an additional 1 2 minutes to melt the crumbled feta cheese.
4. Slide from the skillet to a plate. Season with salt and freshly ground black pepper.

Nutritional Information
- Protein : 20.8 g
- Fat : 26g
- Fiber : 1.5g
- Calories :353

Fluffy Flax Waffles With Turkey Sausage

Servings: 2 | **Prep:** 10 m | **Style:** American | **Cook:** 15 m

Ingredients
- 1 oz raw (yield after cooking) Turkey Breakfast Sausage
- 1 large Egg (Whole)
- 1/16 cup Coconut Milk Unsweetened
- 1/2 tsp Vanilla Extract
- 1/2 tbsp Canola Vegetable Oil
- 1/4 cup Organic 100% Whole Ground Golden Flaxseed Meal
- 1/2 oz Vanilla Whey Protein
- 1 1/2 tsps Sucralose Based Sweetener (Sugar Substitute)
- 1/4 tsp Baking Powder (Straight Phosphate, Double Acting)
- 1/16 tsp Nutmeg (Ground)
- 1/16 tsp Salt

- 1/4 cup Sugar Free Maple Flavored Syrup

Directions
- Brown sausage in a skillet over medium-high heat until cooked through. Remove excess fat by placing on a paper towel and set aside.
- While the sausage is cooking, preheat a non-stick waffle maker. Spray wells with non-stick spray just before pouring in the batter.
- Combine the egg, 1 Tbsp coconut milk, vanilla and oil in a small bowl. Mix thoroughly with a fork for about 1 minute. Add the flax meal, protein powder, granular sugar substitute, baking powder, nutmeg and salt. Mix thoroughly for 1-2 minutes.
- Pour the batter into the waffle maker (it should fill 4 regular 1/2 -inch waffle slots). Otherwise, simply fill with batter according to your waffle maker instructions. For Belgium waffles this recipe makes 2 1/2 squares.
- Cook for 3-5 minutes until golden brown and set. Or follow your waffle maker instructions. Serve with sugar-free pancake syrup and sausage. These waffles freeze well. Reheat in a toaster for 1-2 minutes.

Nutritional Information
- Protein : 32.6 g
- Fat : 36.6g
- Fiber : 16.4g
- Calories :540

Fluffy Flax Waffles

Servings: 2 | **Prep:** 5 m | **Style:** American | **Cook:** 10 m

Ingredients
- 1/8 cup Coconut Milk Unsweetened
- 2 large Eggs (Whole)
- 1 tbsp Canola Vegetable Oil
- 1 tsp Vanilla Extract
- 1/2 cup Organic 100% Whole Ground Golden Flaxseed Meal
- 1 oz Vanilla Whey Protein
- 1/2 tsp Baking Powder (Straight Phosphate, Double Acting)
- 1 tbsp Sucralose Based Sweetener (Sugar Substitute)
- 1/8 tsp Nutmeg (Ground)
- 1/8 tsp Salt

Directions
1. Preheat a non-stick waffle maker. Spray wells with non-stick spray just before pouring in the batter.
2. Combine 2 Tbsp coconut milk, eggs, oil and vanilla in a small bowl. Mix thoroughly with a fork for about 1 minute.
3. Add the flax meal, protein powder, baking powder, granular sugar substitute, nutmeg and salt. Mix thoroughly for 1-2 minutes.
4. Pour 1/2 of batter into the waffle maker (it should fill 4 waffle slots). Otherwise, simply fill with batter according to your waffle maker then equally divide the cooked waffles into two servings once cooked.
5. Cook for 3-5 minutes until golden brown and set. Or follow your waffle maker instructions.
6. Serve with a pad of butter and sugar-free pancake syrup. If you are in Phase 2 or higher add fresh berries!

Nutritional Information
- Protein : 22.2 g
- Fat : 22.5g
- Fiber : 8.4g
- Calories :323

French Quesadillas

Servings: 4 | **Prep:** 10 m | **Style:** American | **Cook**: 5 m

Ingredients
- 3 oz boneless, cooked Fresh Ham
- 1 medium (approx 2-1/2 per lb) Pears
- 4 tortillas Low Carb Tortillas
- 4 oz Brie Cheese
- 1/4 cup sliced Almonds

Directions
1. Preheat oven to 350°F.
2. Lay tortillas flat onto a sheet pan. Layer onto half of each tortilla the pear, ham, Brie cheese and almonds (in that order).
3. Fold the tortilla over and bake for 5 minutes; cut in half and enjoy immediately.

Nutritional Information
- Protein : 16.3 g
- Fat : 15.4g
- Fiber : 6.1g
- Calories :245

French Toast Casserole

Servings: 4 | **Prep:** 45 m | **Style:** American | **Cook**: 80 m

Ingredients

- 14 large Eggs (Whole)
- 10 tbsps Unsalted Butter Stick
- 3 tbsps Xylitol
- 1 cup Organic High Fiber Coconut Flour
- 1 1/2 tsps Baking Powder (Straight Phosphate, Double Acting)
- 3/4 tsp Salt
- 1 cup Heavy Cream
- 1 cup Coconut Milk Unsweetened
- 1 tsp Cinnamon
- 1/4 tsp Nutmeg (Ground)
- 1/2 cup Sugar Free Maple Flavored Syrup

Directions

It is best but not necessary to make the bread portion of this recipe a day or more ahead (a week in advance works great).

1. Preheat oven to 350°F. Grease a small bread pan (8x4-inches). Set aside.
2. Whisk together 8 eggs, 1 tablespoon xylitol and melted butter in a medium bowl.
3. Sift together the coconut flour, baking powder and 3/4 teaspoon salt. Add to the egg mixture and blend until thickened. Bake for 35-40 minutes until the sides pull away from the pan and are golden brown. Allow to cool in the pan for 10 minutes then transfer to a wire rack to finish cooling; about 30 minutes. If baking in advance, once cool, place in an airtight container or zip top bag and refrigerate for up to 2 weeks. If using immediately, once cool, break into 1-inch pieces and place in the same pan used to bake the bread or a small casserole dish.
4. In a medium bowl, whisk together 6 eggs, heavy cream, coconut milk (soy milk or water can replace the coconut milk), 2 tablespoons xylitol, cinnamon, nutmeg and a pinch

of salt. Pour over bread and bake for 50 minutes at 350°F until it is set in the center. Serve immediately by dividing into 8 servings and drizzle each serving with 2 teaspoons sugar-free pancake syrup (or about 1/3 cup over the whole casserole).

Nutritional Information
- Protein : 13.8 g
- Fat : 36.4g
- Fiber : 9.8g
- Calories :440

French Toast Loaf

Servings: 10 | **Prep:** 15 m | **Style:** American | **Cook:** 50 m

Ingredients
- Soy Flour
- 3/4 cup Whole Grain Wheat Flour
- 1 1/4 cups Sucralose Based Sweetener (Sugar Substitute)
- 1 1/2 tbsps Cinnamon
- 1 tsp Salt
- 1 tsp Baking Soda
- 1 cup Buttermilk (Reduced Fat, Cultured)
- 1 tbsp Vanilla Extract
- 1/4 tsp Cream Of Tartar
- 6 large Eggs (Whole)

Directions
1. Preheat oven to 350°F. Grease an 8x4 loaf pan; set aside.
2. In a large bowl, whisk soy flour, whole wheat flour, sugar substitute, cinnamon, salt and baking soda.

3. In another bowl, combine buttermilk, yolks and vanilla. Pour into dry ingredients and using an electric mixer on low speed, beat until smooth.
4. In another bowl, beat whites and cream of tartar with an electric mixer on high speed until medium peaks form, about 4 minutes. Using a rubber spatula, fold whites into batter in three additions. Pour batter into prepared pan and smooth top.
5. Bake 45-50 minutes until golden and a toothpick inserted in center comes out clean. Cool on wire rack for 5 minutes.
6. Invert pan, remove loaf and cut into 10 slices. Serve with warm sugar free maple syrup or fruit preserves.

Nutritional Information
- Protein : 10 g
- Fat : 5.7g
- Fiber : 2.9g
- Calories :156

Frittata Lorraine

Servings: 6 | **Prep**: 20 m | **Style:** American | **Cook:** 10 m

Ingredients
- 8 large Eggs (Whole)
- 1/4 cup Tap Water
- 1/4 tsp Salt
- 1/4 tsp Black Pepper
- 1 small Onion
- 1 cup shredded Gruyere Cheese
- 4 medium slice (yield after cooking) Bacon

Directions

1. Heat a 10-inch nonstick ovenproof skillet over medium-high heat. Add bacon and sauté until it begins to crisp, 3 to 5 minutes. Add white onion and sauté until soft, about 5 minutes.
2. Whisk eggs, water, salt, and pepper in a medium bowl. Add egg mixture and cheese to skillet; cook until eggs are set on bottom but top remains slightly runny, about 5 minutes.
3. Heat broiler to high. Transfer skillet to oven and broil until eggs are set and golden, about 2 minutes. Cut into wedges and serve.

Nutritional Information
- Protein : 15.9 g
- Fat : 14.4g
- Fiber : 0.2g
- Calories :204

Garden Frittata

Servings: 4 | **Prep:** 15 m | **Style:** American | **Cook:** 20 m

Ingredients
- 5 whole Mushroom Pieces and Stems
- 2 leeks Leeks
- 1/4 head large (6-7" dia) Cauliflower
- 2 tbsps Basil
- 1/2 tsp Rosemary (Dried)
- 3 tbsps Parmesan Cheese (Grated)
- 8 large Eggs (Whole)
- 3 tbsps Extra Virgin Olive Oil

Directions
1. Preheat broiler.

2. Heat oil in a medium ovenproof skillet over medium heat. Add leeks and cauliflower; sauté until crisp-tender, about 10 minutes. Add mushrooms, cook 5 minutes, until mushrooms begin to give off liquid.
3. Reduce heat to low. Pour eggs into skillet, stirring slightly. Add basil and rosemary, along with salt and pepper to taste. Cook, stirring frequently, until eggs begin to form small curds and set. Add cheese and lightly press into egg mixture with a spatula.
4. Place skillet under broiler; cook until top is set but not brown, about 1 minute. Cool slightly.
5. To remove frittata whole, tip skillet to one side and use a spatula to loosen edges. Slide onto a serving platter; cut into quarters and serve.

Nutritional Information
- Protein : 14.8 g
- Fat : 20.7g
- Fiber : 1.2g
- Calories :262

Giant Zucchini Pancake

Servings: 4 | **Prep**: 15 m | **Style:** American | **Cook:** 20 m

Ingredients
- 1 lb Baby Zucchini
- 4 slice (1 oz) Havarti Cheese
- 1/3 cup Whole Grain Soy Flour
- 1/3 cup Parsley
- 2 large Eggs (Whole)
- 1/2 tsp Salt
- 1/4 tsp Black Pepper

- 2 tbsps Extra Virgin Olive Oil

Directions
1. Preheat oven to 350°F.
2. Place grated zucchini in a colander and press to drain any excess liquid. Pat zucchini dry with a paper towel.
3. Beat eggs in a large bowl. Stir in cheese, soy flour, parsley, salt and pepper. Add zucchini to cheese mixture. Stir to combine well.
4. In a 10-inch ovenproof skillet, heat oil over medium heat until it shimmers. Add pancake mixture and press down to spread, forming an even layer. Cook 4 minutes or until bottom is set.
5. Transfer skillet to oven; bake 12 15 minutes until middle is just set.
6. Remove from oven and let cool slightly. Cut into wedges and serve crispy side up.

Nutritional Information
- Protein : 13.3 g
- Fat : 21.3g
- Fiber : 2g
- Calories :270

Green Bell Pepper Filled With Creamy Eggs And Spinach

Servings: 1 | **Prep:** 5 m | **Style:** American | **Cook:** 5 m

Ingredients
- 1/2 medium (approx 2-3/4" long, 2-1/2" dia) Green Peppers
- 1 tbsp Extra Virgin Olive Oil
- 1 cup Baby Spinach

- 2 large Eggs (Whole)
- 1 oz Pepper Jack Cheese

Directions
1. Cut bell pepper in half. Slice small slice off the bottom so it will stand up right. Place in a pan with a small amount of water and steam over medium heat until the pepper is tender. Set aside on a serving plate.
2. Sauté 1 cup spinach in a small amount of oil until wilted, add eggs and cheese. Cook until eggs are barely set with a creamy texture (do not over cook) and season with salt and freshly ground black pepper.
3. Spoon the egg mixture into the pepper and serve immediately.

Nutritional Information
- Protein : 19.7 g
- Fat : 32.7g
- Fiber : 2.2g
- Calories :396

Ham And Cheese Roll-Ups

Servings: 6 | **Prep:** 15 m | **Style:** American

Ingredients
- 6 thin slice (approx 4-1/2" x 2-1/2" x 1/8") Fresh Ham
- 6 slice (1 oz) Swiss Cheese
- 6 spears Pickles
- 2 tbsps Real Mayonnaise
- 2 tbsps Dijon Mustard

Directions

1. Trim ham, cheese and pickles to equal lengths. Lay out ham slices, top with cheese slices.
2. Combine mayo and mustard; spread onto cheese. Lay pickle in center and roll up tightly. Cut into bite-sized pieces.

Nutritional Information
- Protein : 14.1 g
- Fat : 13.9g
- Fiber : 0.4g
- Calories :198

www.ingramcontent.com/pod-product-compliance
Lightning Source LLC
Chambersburg PA
CBHW071439070526
44578CB00001B/141